ABC OF LABOUR CARE

ABC OF LABOUR CARE

Edited by

GEOFFREY CHAMBERLAIN

Emeritus Professor of Obstetrics and Gynaecology,
Singleton Hospital, Swansea

PHILIP STEER

Professor of Obstetrics and Consultant Obstetrician,
Imperial College School of Medicine, Chelsea and Westminster Hospital, London

LUKE ZANDER

Senior Lecturer, Department of General Practice and Primary Care,
Guy's, King's and St. Thomas' Hospitals Medical Schools, London

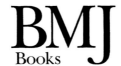

© BMJ Books, 1999
BMJ Books is an imprint of the BMJ Publishing Group

First published in 1999
by BMJ Books, BMA House, Tavistock Square,
London WC1H 9JR

British Library Cataloguing in Publication Data

A catalogue record for this book is avaialble from the British Library

ISBN 0-7279-1415-4

Typeset by Apek Typesetters, Nailsea, Bristol BS48 4DJ
Printed and bound by Craft Print Ltd., Singapore

CONTENTS

Preface   ix

1. Place of birth   LUKE ZANDER, GEOFFREY CHAMBERLAIN   1

2. Physiology and Management of normal labour   PHILIP STEER, CAROLINE FLINT   4

3. Assessment of mother and fetus in labour   PHILIP STEER   8

4. Relief of pain   INGER FINDLEY, GEOFFREY CHAMBERLAIN   12

5. Induction   GEOFFREY CHAMBERLAIN, LUKE ZANDER   16

6. Preterm labour and premature rupture of membranes   PHILIP STEER, CAROLINE FLINT   20

7. Labour in special circumstances   GEOFFREY CHAMBERLAIN, PHILIP STEER   24

8. Unusual presentations and positions and multiple pregnancy   GEOFFREY CHAMBERLAIN, PHILIP STEER   28

9. Operative delivery   GEOFFREY CHAMBERLAIN, PHILIP STEER   31

10. Obstetric emergencies   GEOFFREY CHAMBERLAIN, PHILIP STEER   36

11. Care of the newborn in the delivery room   PATRICIA HAMILTON   40

L'Envoi   45

Index   47

PREFACE

Many of us who qualified before 1990 would be surprised and probably pleased to see what goes on in a labour ward now. The changes in the subject and its application have been massive not only in science but in attitudes and working practices. Evidence based medicine is becoming more important in the care of the pregnant and labouring mother, while the shift of emphasis from obstetrics to midwifery for normal women is continuing. Among the major changes in the last ten years is the wish for the women themselves to have a greater say in decision making and choice of procedures. Generally, if what a mother wants to do in labour is common sense and provided it does not put mother or fetus in danger, she should be encouraged to do it by any attending professionals.

These changes are reflected in this volume. It is based on a series of articles in the BMJ earlier in the year, written by a team of two obstetricians, a general practitioner, a midwife, an anaesthetist and a neonatal paediatrician, recognising that the care of women in labour is a multi-disciplinary task and that the more each worker understands of the role of all team members, the better the results.

This book has chapters by named authors and all are grateful to the staff they work with in their various hospital and community units. Professor Chamberlain is particularly grateful to his secretary Mrs Caron McColl who interpreted the many drafts, and to the midwifery and nursing staff of the Delivery Suite and Special Care Baby Unit of Singleton Hospital, Swansea from where he is also glad to acknowledge help from the ultrasonographers and the Medical Photographer, Mr Douglas Neil. At the BMJ, Julia Thompson catalysed the production of the weekly articles with tact and skill while Anthea Wilkie produced excellent artwork that enhanced the script, and Mary Banks turned them into a book. We are grateful to all of them.

Any opinions are those of the authors; we welcome correspondence from readers to the Senior Editor.

Geoffrey Chamberlain   Philip Steer   Luke Zander
Swansea   London   London

1999

CONTRIBUTORS

Geoffrey Chamberlain
Emeritus Professor of Obstetrics and Gynaecology, Singleton Hospital, Swansea

Inger Findley
Consultant Obstetric Anaesthetist, St George's Hospital, London

Caroline Flint
Honorary Professor, Thames Valley University, London
Independent Midwife, London

Patricia Hamilton
Consultant Neonatologist, St George's Hospital, London

Philip Steer
Professor of Obstetrics and Consultant Obstetrician, Imperial College School of
Medicine, Chelsea and Westminster Hospital, London

Luke Zander
Senior Lecturer, Department of General Practice and Primary Care, Guy's King's
and St Thomas' Hospitals Medical Schools, London

1 Place of birth

Luke Zander, Geoffrey Chamberlain

The management of childbirth is continuously evolving, reflecting changes in clinical, psychological, and social factors. In the past 50 years there have been dramatic falls in perinatal and maternal mortality, a steady increase in the amount of technological intervention in the management of labour, and a change in the roles of members of the maternity care team.

Over the past 60 years the proportion of births at home has fallen markedly from 80% in 1930 to 1% in 1990, but in the past eight years the proportion has begun to rise again. Some studies suggest that 10-14% of women would choose this option if given the opportunity. A similar trend has been seen in all Western countries except the Netherlands, where, in 1995, 32% of births still occurred in the home.

When considering how a birth is to be conducted, attention must be given to both risks and benefits. The debate over the place of birth raises many fundamental questions about the general management of labour, patients' satisfaction, and women's rights to choose their form of care. Much professional and lay discussion has taken place on many aspects of pregnancy care, brought into focus by the Department of Health's 1993 report *Changing Childbirth*, which indicated the way the maternity services may develop. Safety is the foundation of good maternity care but this must take into account the emotional as well as the physical wellbeing of mother and baby.

Care settings

Home
The home is the place for the practice of midwifery, not obstetrics, and the principal provider of care will be the midwife. The home is therefore appropriate for mothers with a low risk of complications. If any form of intervention is needed the appropriate course of action will almost inevitably be to transfer the woman or baby to the nearest suitable maternity unit. This is irrespective of the competence of the professionals present, for the home is not a suitable setting for undertaking obstetric procedures. It has long been assumed that hospital provides a safer environment for women at low risk as well as the high risk mothers. This assumption, however, is not evidence based.

Free standing general practitioner maternity units
The number of independent general practitioner maternity units has declined markedly over the past 30 years. They are usually much appreciated by women because of their informal approach and accessibility, and attempts at closure often provoke strong opposition. The level of care lies somewhere

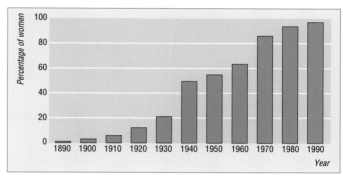

Percentage of women giving birth in United Kingdom in 1890-1990 who delivered in hospital

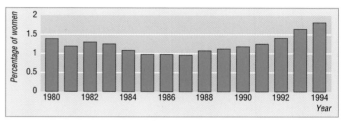

Percentage of women giving birth in England and Wales in 1980-94 who delivered at home

---

Objectives of good labour care
- To provide a safe outcome for the mother and baby with the minimum of avoidable complications
- To make the birth experience as satisfying as possible for the mother and her family
- To make optimal use of the available resources

"**The woman must be the focus of maternity care. She should be able to feel she is in control of what is happening to her and able to make decisions about her care based on her needs, having discussed matters fully with the professionals involved.**"
From *Changing Childbirth*

Is hospital really the safest place to deliver?*
- A statistical association between the increase in the proportion of hospital births and the fall in crude perinatal mortality seems unlikely to be the result of cause and effect
- No evidence exists to support the claim that a hospital is the safest place for women to have normal births
- The policy of closing small obstetric units on the grounds of safety is unsupported by available evidence

*Conclusions from *Where to be Born*, published by the National Perinatal Epidemiology Unit, 1994

Reasons that women choose home birth*
To avoid unnecessary intervention	31%
To be on familiar territory so as to be more relaxed and in control	25%
Previous home birth	11%
Wish to be in a familiar setting in which they feel relaxed	10%
Fear of hospital setting	10%
To have a continuing relationship with midwife	4%

*Data from National Birthday Trust's 1994 home births survey (see *Home Births* in key references box)

between home and the specialist unit. If safety is to be maintained, criteria for selection and protocols for care need to be established, ideally by a multidisciplinary group representing all those engaged in the provision of care.

Integrated general practitioner units

A major advantage of having a general practitioner unit closely linked to an obstetric unit is the immediate availability of specialist skills if required. Such proximity, however, might discourage the involvement of general practitioners and might also change the ambience of the care provided so that it becomes more like that of the specialist unit.

Most general practice units report low perinatal mortality and low rates of intervention compared with the national rates derived from total populations. This is partly because the women delivering at these units will have a low risk of complications.

Midwifery led units

Midwifery led units, either independent from or attached to a specialist obstetric unit, are becoming more common and reflect the fact that midwives provide care at 75% of deliveries. If specialist obstetric or neonatal help is required, the midwife is responsible for seeking it. Giving midwives organisational and clinical responsibility indicates recognition of their professional status and expertise. It is possible that such units will be the models for most delivery units of the future, providing continuity of care throughout pregnancy, labour, and the puerperium.

Consultant led units

Over 90% of labour care is currently provided in consultant led units. Smaller units (under 2500 deliveries a year) may in future have problems with staffing and recognition of their junior obstetric, paediatric, or anaesthetic posts for training purposes. With the expanding role of the midwife and the desire for continuity of care, a large part of a specialist's clinical work will be supervisory and acting as a point of referral for women identified antenatally or during labour as needing specialist services. Hence obstetricians will act in a way that is more like that of specialists in other branches of medicine.

Dealing with emergencies

Acute, unforeseen emergencies can occur to the mother or fetus at any time during labour or to either after delivery. It is therefore essential that wherever birth takes place adequate arrangements are available to deal with emergencies; midwives and general practitioners must be appropriately trained. In hospital, staff and equipment can speedily be summoned; this is not so at home or in a freestanding unit. The flying squad is no longer a viable option for it removes essential staff from the hospital. It will be the paramedics who help at emergencies away from hospital. They are trained to provide the immediate care for all emergencies (including obstetrics) in most areas.

General practitioners and labour care

General practitioners may provide labour care at home or in the general practitioner maternity unit. The number of general practitioners actively involved in labour care has declined markedly over the past 30-40 years. Whereas in 1965 about 50% of all births took place under a general practitioner's care, in 1994 delivery by a general practitioner was reported in only 800 out of 604 300 women. General practitioners are uncertain about their responsibility and role in labour care and how to

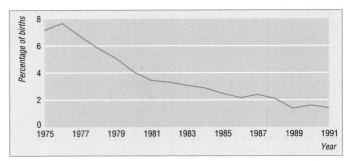

Percentage of births in England and Wales in 1975-91 in a freestanding general practitioner unit

---

Deliveries in freestanding general practitioner units, England and Wales

1975	43 862 deliveries
1995	9 374 deliveries

Recent data from two freestanding midwifery delivery units

	No of bookings (births)	No (%) of transfers			
		Before birth	During labour	Postnatally	
				Mother	Baby
Aberdare (Sep 1997- Aug 1998)	249 (209)	40 (16)*	20 (10)†	3 (1)†	2 (1)†
Crowborough (Apr 1997- Mar 1998)	331 (179)	109 (33)*	17 (9)†	1	0

*Percentage of bookings; †percentage of births.

Reasons that women choose a hospital birth*

Safety	84%
Previous hospital birth	6%

*Data from National Birthday Trust's 1994 home births survey (see *Home Births* in key references box)

Special tertiary care centres will always be needed for particular obstetric and neonatal problems. Consideration must be given to how these centres can best be integrated into the overall provision of services

---

Reasons for changes in general practitioners' involvement in labour care

- Perceived lack of expertise
- Fear of litigation
- Changes in the organisation of out of hours cover
- Unacceptable encroachment on off duty hours
- Inadequate remuneration

respond to a woman's request for home birth. To clarify the position, the General Medical Services Committee recently spelt out the duties of general practitioners in labour care.

General practitioners can be involved in labour care at one or more of four levels. Many general practitioners feel reluctant to become involved because of a perceived risk of litigation. Such concern relates not only to their own level of competence but also to the care provided by the midwife.

Four levels of potential general practitioner involvement in labour care

- Providing the necessary information and advice
- Referring women for further care to the appropriate professional (midwife, obstetrician, or another general practitioner)
- Being present during labour to provide psychosocial support for the woman and non-specialist support for the midwife
- Providing practical labour care in a general practitioner maternity unit. This would require a higher level of training (only general practitioners undertaking this type of work can be called "general practitioner obstetricians")

Lead professonals

Changing Childbirth recommended that for each pregnant woman there would be a clearly identified lead professional responsible for ensuring that the woman received the appropriate care. This will usually be a midwife. Good communication between the lead professional and other members of the maternity care team is essential so that each can contribute appropriately to the overall care.

Women centred care

In whatever setting birth takes place, every effort should be made to ensure that the woman is made to feel physically and psychologically as comfortable as possible. She should perceive herself to be in control of what is happening and be able to make decisions about her care, having had full discussions with the professionals involved. If this is to be achieved certain requirements need to be instituted (see box).

Conclusions

Childbirth is one of life's major events. The way in which it is experienced will have very significant and long term effects on the mother. It is the responsibility of all those involved in the provision of care to achieve a balance between scientific objectivity and a concern for the woman's wishes.

The future lies with an expansion of midwife led delivery units in hospitals with birth rooms, and with an early return home after delivery. Doctors will still be needed when progress varies from normal.

The graphs showing percentages of hospital and home births are based on data from the Office of Populations, Censuses, and Surveys. Gillian Halksworth-Smith of the University of Glamorgan and staff of the Crowborough birthing centre provided the data for the table on the second page.

Duties of general practitioners in labour care*

- To provide impartial advice regarding the availability of local services
- To discuss the available options in a way that the woman can make an informed choice
- To arrange for the provision of care

*As defined by the General Medical Services Committee

Legal responsibilities of general practitioners in labour care*

- General practitioners are responsible only for their own acts or omissions
- Midwives are accountable for their actions and decisions regardless of where they work
- General practitioners do not have to attend a birth at home unless requested to do so by the midwife (regardless of whether they have agreed to provide maternity care for that woman)
- If a general practitioner undertakes labour care and a mishap occurs, at litigation the general practitioner would be judged by the standards of a colleague of similar skills and training, not those of a specialist obstetrician

*According to Maternity Task Group of the Royal College of General Practitioners, 1995

> The lead professional is responsible for ensuring that the woman receives appropriate care and that all the services provided by her different carers are fully coordinated. The lead professional will usually be a midwife

---

Requirements of women centred care*

- An appropriate range of options of care need to be provided
- Women need to be informed of the options available
- Women need to be able to establish a relationship with their care providers so that their views and preferences can be discussed
- A woman's preferences need to be recorded in her records so that they can be acted on appropriately by those providing her care even if they have not met her before
- Attention needs to be given to the physical design of the surroundings and the availability of relevant facilities, such as water pools or birth aids

*According to *Changing Childbirth*

Key references

- Campbell R, MacFarlane A. *Where to be born?* Oxford: National Perinatal Epidemiology Unit, 1994.
- Chamberlain G, Wraight A, Crowley P. *Home births.* Carnford: Pergamon Press, 1997.
- Department of Health. *Changing childbirth.* London: HMSO, 1993, 1994.
- General Services Medical Council. *General practitioners and intrapartum care—interim guidance.* London: BMJ Publishing, 1997.
- *Statistical bulletin. NHS maternity statistics England 1989-1995.* London: Stationery Office, 1997.
- Maternity Task Group of the Royal College of General Practitioners. The role of the general practitioner in maternity care. London: RCGP, 1995. (Occasional paper No 72.)
- Welsh Office. *Health evidence bulletin. Maternal and child health.* Cardiff: NHS Wales, 1998.

2 Physiology and management of normal labour

Philip Steer, Caroline Flint

Labour is more difficult in humans than in most other mammals. Our ancestors, the Australopithecines, adopted the upright posture about five million years ago. Natural selection produced a smaller pelvis, which more efficiently transmits forces from the hind legs to the spine. About 1.5 million years ago brain size began to increase (probably associated with improved social integration and later with the language instinct), with the result that the head of the human fetus at term now takes up most of the available space in the mother's pelvis.

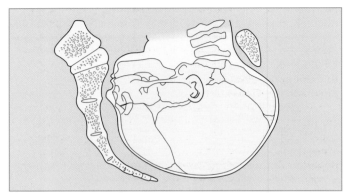

Longitudinal view of fetal head in the pelvis showing how little room there is

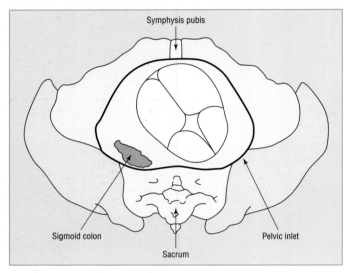

Horizontal view of engagement in left occipito-anterior position

It was probably only because of the development of rotation of the head during labour some 300 000 years ago that the system of human birth works at all. The fetal head usually engages in the occipito-transverse position and rotates to occipito-anterior as it passes through the pelvis, allowing the shoulders to engage in the pelvic brim in the transverse position. Once the head is born, the shoulders rotate into the anterior-posterior position, which facilitates their delivery.

The normal uterus is spontaneously contractile, and it is largely the progesterone secreted from the placenta that suppresses activity of the uterus during pregnancy, keeping the fetus in the uterus. In addition, the cervix remains firm and non-compliant. At term, changes occur in the cervix that make it softer, and uterine contractions become more frequent and regular. The precise mechanisms of these changes remain obscure. Changes in the ratio of oestrogen to progesterone, fetal steroid secretion, and changes in the tension of the uterine wall as the fetus grows probably all play a part. Evidence is increasing that the long term interests of the fetus are best served by it being large at birth. However, this represents a problem for the mother, as some women experience long term pelvic damage from delivering large babies. This conflict between the interests of the baby and the mother is probably the reason that the duration of pregnancy is variable. The mother gives birth more easily if the baby is premature, but the baby survives best if born at term and larger.

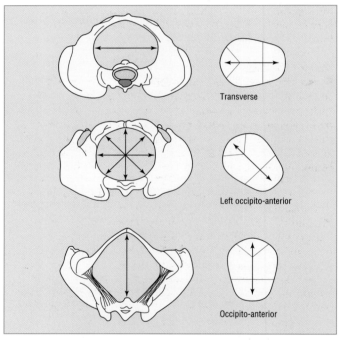

Rotation of fetal head as it descends through the pelvis. The maximum diameter of the head matches that of the pelvis at each level (maximum diameters are indicated by an arrow)

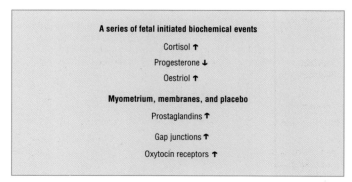

Factors implicated in the onset of labour

Stages of labour

Labour can be divided into three stages, which are unequal in length. The fundamental change underlying the process of the first stage is progressive dilatation of the cervix. This gives rise to the familiar symptoms and signs of labour. The cervix is richly supplied with nerve endings, and as it starts to dilate, this gives rise to the characteristic pain of labour. In addition, the plug of viscous mucus that has protected against the ingress of bacteria during pregnancy often emerges as a show. The dilatation of the cervix reduces the support for the fetal amniotic membranes, which bulge through the cervix, and often the rupture of these membranes can be the initiating phenomenon of active labour.

Under optimal circumstances regular uterine contractions are prompted by the development of contacts between cells considered to be sites of low resistance. These gap junctions are sites of low electrical resistance which allow the passage of depolarisation waves from one muscle cell to another across the uterus. Ideally the process coincides with the ripening of the cervix. If the contractions start or the membranes rupture before the cervix is properly ripe, the process is stimulated by the release of prostaglandins from the membranes and the uterine decidua. Then labour has to pass through a latent phase during which the cervix dilates only very slowly. This can be very demoralising for the mother and increases the risk of infection during labour.

Monitoring labour

Progress in the latent phase of labour is assessed with the Bishop score. The cervix should change at a minimum of one Bishop score point an hour if labour is to end within a reasonable time (only 20% of women move more slowly than this). A score of 11 indicates the onset of the active phase of labour, during which the average rate of cervical dilatation in women in their first labour is 1 cm/h. In parous women the cervix dilates faster—on average 1.6 cm/h.

An important development in the management of labour was the introduction of the partogram. First developed by Hugh Philpott in 1972 to identify abnormally slow labour, the partogram is a graphical representation of the changes that occur in labour, including cervical dilatation, fetal heart rate, maternal pulse, blood pressure, and temperature; it also shows a numerical record of features such as urine output and the volume and type of intravenous infusions (including oxytocin drips). It is therefore possible at a glance to identify deviations from normal in any of these variables.

Three stages of labour

- First: from the onset of labour to full dilatation (commonly lasts 8-12 hours in a first labour, 3-8 hours in subsequent labours)
- Second: from full dilatation of the cervix to delivery of the baby (commonly lasts 1-2 hours in a first labour, 0.5-1 hour in subsequent labours)
- Third: from delivery of the baby to the delivery of the placenta (commonly lasts up to an hour if physiological, 5-15 minutes if actively managed)

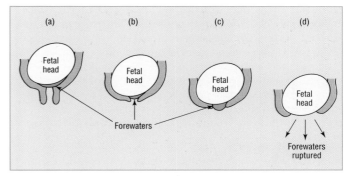

Dilatation of the cervix: *(a)* cervix not taken up or dilated in late pregnancy; *(b)* cervix 1 cm dilated; *(c)* cervix 2-3 cm dilated with a bag of membranes bulging; *(d)* cervix 5 cm dilated with the membranes ruptured and amniotic fluid escaping

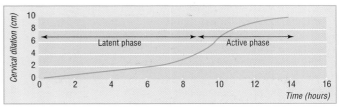

Latent and active phases of labour in a primiparous woman

Bishop score for assessing cervical ripeness

	0	1	2	3
Cervical length (cm)	1	1 or 2	<1	Fully taken up
Cervical dilatation (cm)	0	1 or 2	3 or 4	≥5
Cervical consistency	Firm	Medium	Soft	NA
Position of cervix	Posterior	Central	Anterior	NA
Station of presenting part (cm above ischial spines)	3	2	1 or 0	Below spines

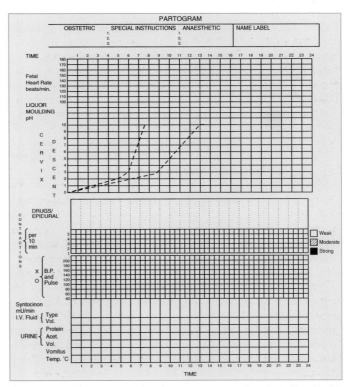

Partogram: the broken lines show expected progress of cervical dilatation in multiparous (left) and primiparous (right) women

It is difficult to predict how a labour will progress; we cannot predict the likely strength and frequency of uterine contractions, the extent to which the cervix will soften and dilate, and the extent of moulding of the fetal head. Equally, we cannot know beforehand whether the complex fetal rotation needed for an efficient labour will take place properly. For all these reasons, antenatal pelvimetry has not proved to be a useful predictor, except among those who have had traumatic damage—for example, a fracture of the pelvis.

Oxygen supply

The oxygen supply is reduced during labour because contractions interfere with the flow of oxygenated maternal blood to the placenta. However, the fetus normally adapts well to this. The fetal circulation is unaffected by contractions (as the fetus is enclosed within the uterus), unless there is cord entanglement with compression. The normal oxygen tension in the fetal blood before labour is about 4 kPa. During labour it falls to about 3 kPa. However, redistribution of the flow within the fetus to protect the vital organs—such as the heart and brain—means that a healthy fetus copes well with this stress.

Delivery of placenta

Once the baby is born, the uterus continues to contract strongly and can now retract, decreasing markedly in size. This shears off the placenta from the uterine wall. If the placenta is allowed to be delivered with normal contractions (sometimes called "physiological management"), this can take up to an hour. Use of an oxytocic drug speeds this process fourfold and reduces average blood loss by about 50%. A recent study published in the *Lancet* showed that in a large randomised controlled trial only 6.8% of women receiving active (drug) management had significant bleeding, compared with 16.5% receiving physiological management.

Use of drugs

Oxytocic drugs should be given with the birth of the anterior shoulder. The use of antenatal ultrasound screening has virtually eliminated the possibility of giving the oxytocic before the birth of an undiagnosed second twin. Syntocinon is the most used oxytocic known to be effective; the addition of ergometrine may reduce blood loss even further but can cause serious hypertension in susceptible women—for example, those with pre-eclampsia. Because of the speed with which the uterus retracts after stimulation with an oxytocic, the placenta should be removed by controlled cord traction as soon as it is perceived to have separated from the uterine wall.

Support for mother

As most labours are spontaneous and end with a normal delivery, the main purpose of the birth attendant (usually a midwife) is to provide support for the mother and her partner in labour and to monitor the process for abnormality. The birth attendant therefore needs to understand both the physical processes and the emotional needs of the mother.

It is difficult for a nulliparous woman to understand the sensations (including sometimes severe pain) that she will experience during childbirth until they actually occur. The birth attendant therefore needs to interpret the woman's sensations for her—for example, explaining that fears that "the baby is stuck" and "my perineum is going to split apart" are normal and do not necessarily indicate an abnormality.

Some women need a quietly supportive approach; others need boisterous encouragement (especially while pushing in the

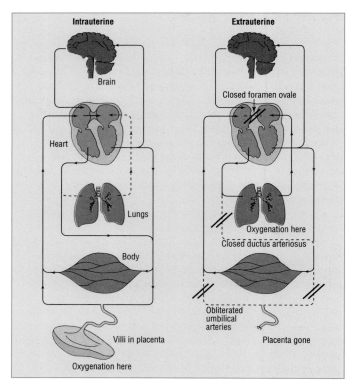

Essential changes between intrauterine circulation and extrauterine circulation (the bypasses that close at or soon after birth are marked with parallel lines)

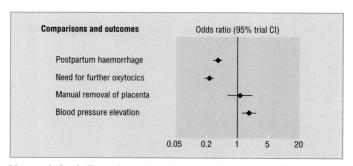

Meta-analysis of effects of prophylactic oxytocic drugs in blood loss during third stage of labour

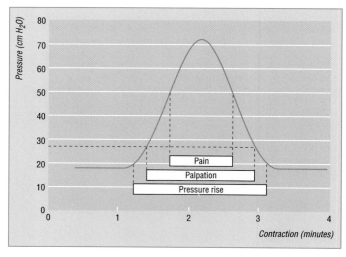

Pressure recording of a uterine contraction in the later first stage of labour (note differentials of pressure rise with objective palpation of contractions and pain felt by the mother)

second stage). Sensitivity and experience are needed to match the type of support with the needs of the mother.

Delivery positions

Because women in labour are in pain they often feel the need to move around a great deal. It is therefore helpful to provide an environment in which the woman can vary her position at will—for example, soft mats and bean bags on the floor, cushions, or birth pools. The woman should be encouraged to deliver in whichever position she feels comfortable, providing that this does not affect the fetus significantly. Some women like standing or squatting, but the most commonly used position is lying propped up on a bed; the only position that should routinely be proscribed is the supine position (that is, with the woman flat on her back). This often causes caval compression, restricting venous return from the legs, and can result in the supine hypotension syndrome, leading to fetal and maternal hypoxia. If the supine position has to be used—for example, for vacuum or forceps delivery—a wedge should be placed under the mother's buttocks and lower back to tilt the uterus away from the inferior vena cava.

Other roles of birth attendant

The value of physical guidance of the fetus by the attendant at a normal birth is controversial. The HOOP ("hands on or poised") study, in which control of the emergence of the head and shoulders is being compared with entirely spontaneous birth is still under way.

   After the birth, the birth attendant should be vigilant for any signs of haemorrhage or infection.

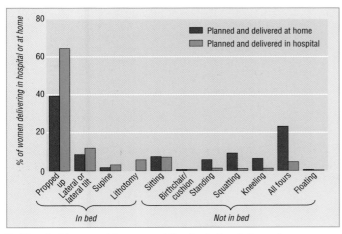

Positions in labour used by women delivering in hospital or at home

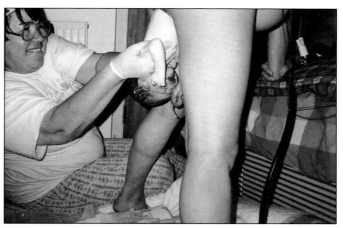

Delivery in a standing position

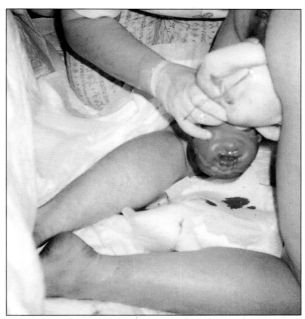

Delivery in hands and knees position

Conclusions

- The approach to the management of labour in Britain is increasingly liberal
- The midwife, a professional in her own right, now has greater autonomy and responsibility
- Many of the older, restrictive measures on feeding, walking, and position for delivery are not effective, efficient, or necessary

The diagram showing essential changes between intrauterine and extrauterine circulation is adapted from Chamberlain (*Lecture notes—obstetrics.* 7th ed. Oxford: Blackwell Science, 1997). The line drawing showing the results of meta-analysis of effects of prophylactic oxytocic drugs is adapted from Prendeville W, Elbourne D (*Cochrane Pregnancy and Childbirth Database* (1995, issue 2)). The graph showing positions in labour used by women is adapted from *Home Births* (National Birthday Trust survey, 1994).

Key references

- Barker D. Fetal origins of coronary heart disease. *BMJ* 1995; 311:171-4.
- Philpott RH. Graphic records in labour. *BMJ* 1972;iv:163-5.
- Rogers J, Wood J, McCandlish R, Ayers S, Truesdale A, Elbourne D. Active versus expectant management of third stage of labour: the Hinchingbrooke randomised controlled trial. *Lancet* 1998; 351:693-9.
- Liu D, Fairweather D. *Labour ward manual.* Oxford: Butterworth-Heinemann, 1991.
- Whittle M. The management and monitoring of normal labour. In: Chamberlain G, ed. *Turnbull's obstetrics.* London: Churchill Livingstone, 1995.
- Davies R. The midwife's role in the management of normal labour. In: Chamberlain G, ed. *Turnbull's obstetrics.* London: Churchill Livingstone, 1995.

3 Assessment of mother and fetus in labour

Philip Steer

The management of labour used to be largely expectant—"wait and see" or "never let the sun set twice on a labouring woman," implying that a labour taking up to 48 hours was acceptable. Labours of this length are often emotionally traumatic for women, may hide hazards to the fetus, and are very demanding on staff resources. In the 1960s, '70s, and '80s O'Driscoll and colleagues promoted *active management* of labour for women in their first labour. This management emphasised:

● A policy of non-interference for women not definitely in labour;

● Regular assessment of cervical dilatation;

● Early intervention, with artificial rupture of membranes and infusion of Syntocinon if labour progressed more slowly than 1 cm/h; and

● One to one care with a skilled birth attendant.

Subsequent studies showed that, although this approach reduces the length of labour by a small amount, the only component with a clear benefit in promoting spontaneous vaginal birth is the continuous presence of the birth attendant. Women have declared their intolerance of long labours, however, by increasingly requesting delivery by caesarean section. In many major maternity units in the developed world, the rate of caesarean sections is now 16% or higher. In the United Kingdom this process has been accelerated by the *Changing Childbirth* initiative, which emphasises the importance of maternal preferences.

Commonest monitoring techniques

Currently, the most common recommendations for monitoring progress in labour are measuring the descent of the fetal head and a vaginal examination of cervical dilatation every four hours. The rate of dilatation below which augmentation by Syntocinon infusion is recommended varies from 1 cm/h (the original O'Driscoll recommendation, resulting in augmentation rates in first labours of 40-50%) to 0.5 cm/h (leading to augmentation rates of about 15%). The mother's condition is assessed by repeating blood pressure measurements, recording her temperature, and checking hydration by the volume of urine and ketone concentration in the urine produced. These variables are recorded on a combined flow chart (a partogram).

Electronic fetal heart rate monitoring

The fetal condition is monitored by assessment of the fetal heart rate, either by intermittent auscultation or by continuous electronic monitoring. The former is performed at intervals varying from every 2 hours to every 15 minutes, depending on the circumstances—for example, more frequently if there is meconium staining of the amniotic fluid, or during the second stage. Auscultation is best performed at the end of a contraction, to detect late decelerations (transient decrease in heart rate occurring at or after the end of a uterine contraction), but at this time the fetal heart is often difficult to hear. Use of a portable Doppler fetal heart detector has revolutionised this procedure, making it possible to count the fetal heart rate easily with the woman in any position; there are even waterproof machines for use in birth pools. A fetal heart rate above

Rates of oxytocin augmentation in primiparous women and incidence of caesarean section during labour

	1968	1972	1980
Oxytocin augmentation (%)	11	55	41
Caesarean section (%)	1.2	1.8	1.2

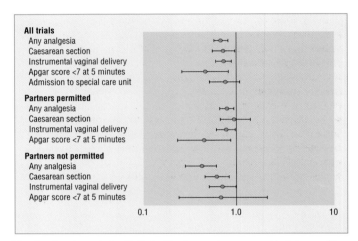

Results of meta-analysis of effect of having partners present in labour (with odds ratios and 95% confidence intervals for various outcomes)

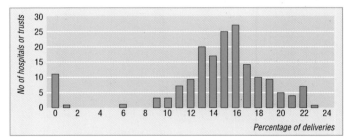

Distribution of percentages of deliveries by caesarean section at different hospitals in England and Wales

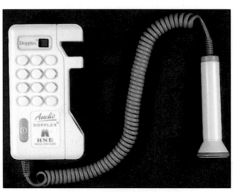

Handheld Doppler fetal heart rate monitor

150 beats/minute or below 110 beats/minute for more than a few minutes requires further investigation by continuous electronic fetal heart rate monitoring. Any slowing of the heart rate by more than 15 beats/minute after contractions is also an indication for electronic monitoring.

Drawbacks

In recent years continuous electronic fetal heart rate monitoring has had a bad press. This is due at least partly to a false expectation that it could reveal all about fetal condition during labour. In fact, it is a good method for screening for umbilical cord compression, fetal hypoxia, and acidosis. It has a high sensitivity for these problems, but the main drawback is its high false positive rate. During the first stage of labour about a fifth of normal fetuses will have a fetal heart rate pattern that is not normal; most abnormalities reflect stress—for example, temporary cord compression or hypoxia—rather than distress.

To reduce unnecessary operative delivery for erroneous suspicions of acidosis, it is essential that electronic fetal heart rate monitoring is supplemented by fetal blood sampling with pH and base deficit measurement. Unfortunately, this technique is time consuming and is therefore used regularly in only about half the maternity units in Britain. Other drawbacks to electronic monitoring are:
- Its unreliability in detecting intrapartum infection, which sometimes causes a fetal tachycardia (most tachycardias, however, are due to maternal fever, common in labour, especially in association with epidural analgesia); and
- Its inability to predict acute trauma, such as shoulder dystocia.

Accepted indications for continuous electronic fetal heart rate monitoring in labour

- At risk features in mothers:
  Diabetes
  Hypertension
  Labour before 34 weeks
  Labour after 42 weeks
- Intermittent monitoring shows:
  Tachycardia >150 beats/minute
  Bradycardia <110 beats/minute
  Slowing of heart beat by >15 beats/minute after contraction
- Meconium staining of liquor

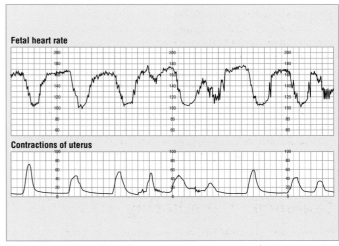

Cardiotocogram showing variable decelerations (transient series of decelerations in heart rate that vary in duration, intensity, and relation to uterine contractions)

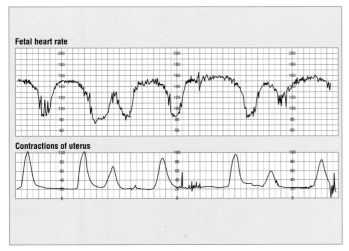

Cardiotocogram showing late decelerations

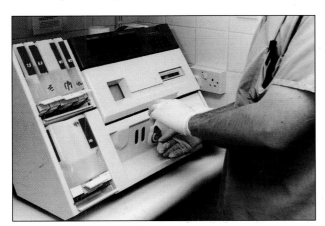

Fetal pH and blood gases analyser

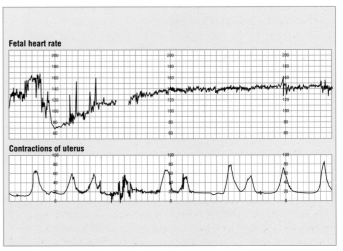

Cardiotocogram showing profound deceleration and loss of beat to beat variation after the woman lay in supine position

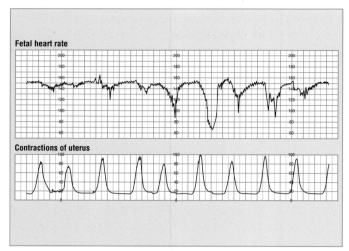

Cardiotocogram showing variable decelerations after oxytocic stimulation

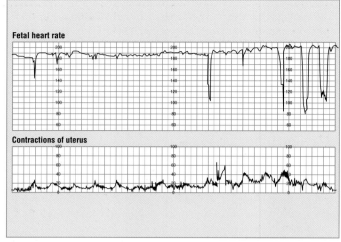

Cardiotocogram showing fetal tachycardia and variable decelerations with maternal fever

A further problem is that the interpretation of fetal heart rate patterns is notoriously subjective. Although specialists can reliably distinguish abnormal from normal patterns, this is much more difficult for beginners, who despite their lack of experience are often overconfident. Even the specialists find some patterns difficult to interpret. Although late decelerations nearly always indicate some degree of hypoxia, fetal reserve is variable, and the ability of the fetus to cope over a period of time can be assessed only with serial blood sampling to give blood gas and pH estimation.

Passage of meconium

The second traditional indicator of fetal distress is the passage of meconium by the fetus during labour. Meconium is the contents of the fetal bowel, and presence of bile acids and salts renders meconium very corrosive. Normal fetuses usually pass meconium only after they have been born. The stimulus for its passage is probably activation of massive sensory input, a part of the "fight, flight, and fright" reaction. Some fetuses pass meconium in response to stress while still *in utero*—most commonly, during labour. The proportion of fetuses passing meconium rises from less than 4% before 34 completed weeks to over 30% at 42 weeks. Having meconium in the amniotic fluid is relatively harmless for the fetus so long as it does not inhale the contaminated liquor. The stimulus for gasping *in utero* is not known but may well include acute hypoxia.

The combination of meconium in the amniotic fluid and gasping leads to the meconium aspiration syndrome, still a cause of neonatal mortality in Britain. The appearance of meconium during labour does not in itself indicate fetal distress as it is often associated with healthy fetuses, so provided the fetal heart rate remains normal, there is no increased likelihood of fetal acidosis. If the fetal heart rate becomes abnormal, however, the potential for meconium aspiration is increased.

New techniques

Several new methods of fetal assessment, such as fetal electrocardiographic wave form analysis, fetal pulse oximetry, and near infrared spectroscopy for assessment of acidosis, are technically difficult to implement. They are still research tools. New microsampling methods of measuring lactate in the fetal blood, however, have the potential for assessing fetal acid base reserve in a way that is simpler, cheaper, and more reliable.

Computerised analysis of fetal heart rate patterns
- Computerised analysis of fetal heart rate patterns in labour is now almost possible, as recent trials of such systems have been encouraging
- Computer based teaching programmes offer a real chance of improving the general standard of interpretation

The combination of meconium staining of the amniotic fluid and a fetal heart rate that clearly indicates hypoxia is probably a sufficient indication for caesarean delivery, even if the fetal pH is normal at that time

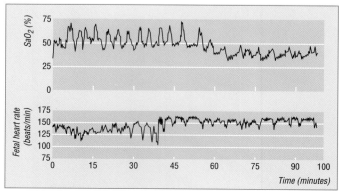

A fetal pulse oximetry recording

Advantages of measuring lactate over pH estimates in fetal blood sampling to detect a hypoxic fetus*

- Less dilatation of the cervix is needed
- Fewer scalp punctures are needed
- Sampling technique is faster
- Less fetal blood is needed (5μl *v* 35μl)

*From Westgren M et al (*Br J Obstet Gynaecol* 1998;105:29-33)

Preventing errors

Confidential inquiries into perinatal death indicate that in 60% of labours there is a preventable element related to incorrect assessment of fetal monitoring. Studies of the causes of perinatal death and cerebral palsy have suggested a 50% and 25% rate respectively of possibly avoidable errors related to fetal monitoring. It seems that there is more to be gained at the moment by improved use of current technology than by trying to implement completely new methods of monitoring.

Leading areas of clinical error

According to data from the confidential inquiry into stillbirths and deaths in infancy for England and Wales 1994-5, the five leading areas of clinical error, in decreasing rank order are:

- Assessment of fetal condition during labour, particularly with regard to the use of electronic fetal heart rate monitoring and fetal blood sampling;
- Recognition of risk during labour;
- Management of labour;
- Assessment of risk factors before labour; and
- Management of delivery.

These were the leading areas found among 873 deaths during labour of normal babies (> 1500 g birth weight). Better care would have improved outcome in 52% of cases and might have done in another 25%.

The data in the table showing rates of oxytocin augmentation and incidence of caesarean section are taken from O'Driscoll K et al (*Obstet Gynaec* 1984;63;485-90). The graph showing results of the meta-analysis is adapted from Thornton J et al (*BMJ* 1994;309:366-9). The graph showing the distribution of caesarean sections is adapted from the *Statistical Bulletin NHS Maternity Statistics* (London: Stationery Office, 1997). The cardiotocograms are adapted from *Fetal Heart Rate Monitoring—A Practical Guide* (Oxford: Oxford University Press, 1993). The fetal pulse oximetry recording is adapted from Johnson et al (*Br J Obstet Gynaecol* 1991;98: 36-41). The graph showing results of infrared spectrometry is adapted from Peebles et al (*Am J Obstet Gynecol* 1992;166:1369-73).

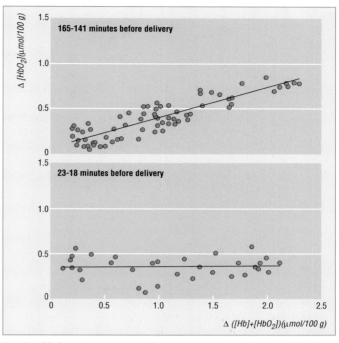

Results of infrared spectrometry. Changes in cerebral oxyhaemoglobin plus deoxyhaemoglobin during first (top) and second (bottom) stages of labour in one fetus. Each point represents a 10 second collection of data during three consecutive contractions. Mean cerebral haemoglobin oxygen saturation, calculated from the least-mean-squares regression, was 35 (±2%) at 165-141 minutes and 1 (±3%) at 23-18 minutes before delivery

Key references

- Department of Health. *Changing childbirth.* London: HMSO, 1992.
- O'Driscoll K, Jackson RJA, Gallagher JT. Prevention of prolonged labour. *BMJ* 1969;ii:477-80.
- O'Driscoll K, Stronge JM, Minogue M. Active management of labour *BMJ* 1973;3:135-7.
- O'Driscoll K, Foley M, MacDonald D. Active management of labour as an alternative to caesarean section for dystocia. *Obstet Gynecol* 1984;63:485-90.
- Westgren M, KrugerK, Ek S, Gunnaralt C, Kublickas M, Naka K, et al. Lactate compared with pH analysis at fetal scalp blood sampling: a prospective randomised study. *Br J Obstet Gynaecol* 1998;105:29-33.
- Spencer J, Ward H. *Intrapartum fetal surveillance.* London: RCOG Press, 1993.
- Ingermarsson J, Ingermarsson H, Spencer J. *Fetal heart rate monitoring. A practical guide.* Oxford: Oxford University Press, 1993.
- *Confidential Enquiry into Stillbirths and Deaths in Infancy.* London: Maternal and Child Health Research Consortium, 1998.

4 Relief of pain

Inger Findley, Geoffrey Chamberlain

Labour is usually painful. Exceptionally, a very few women may not feel pain; others can control their response so as to reduce pain. Most women think that pain is going to be a major part of giving birth. Professionals can help to reduce women's fears by giving precise, accurate, and relevant information beforehand and explaining what pain relief will be available at the place where the woman will be in labour. If a women has plans about the sort of pain relief she wants, these should be discussed in advance with the woman and her partner.

The National Birthday Trust has performed nationwide surveys since the second world war, and the table shows the proportions of women going through labour using various methods of analgesia. Chloroform and trilene are no longer used; pethidine achieved a popularity that is now waning; nitrous oxide is a mainstay; and epidural and spinal methods are increasing in use.

The Trust's 1990 report, *Pain Relief in Labour*, is based on the experiences of over 10 000 women who delivered in the United Kingdom during one week. It is the best source of national statistics on both pharmacological and non-pharmacological analgesics. Much of this article is based on the report; some practices may have changed in the years since the survey—for example, the increased use of epidural and spinal anaesthesia for caesarean section.

Pharmacological methods

Nitrous oxide

Premixed nitrous oxide and oxygen is now provided as Entonox. It is a 50:50 mixture and is available at virtually all places of delivery.

Nitrous oxide is self administered, but women cannot take too much as the flow stops before consciousness is lost. The mixture improves fetal oxygeneration and has a very short half life. About 85% of women find it helpful.

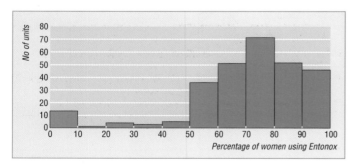

Percentage of women using nitrous oxide by distribution of numbers of labour units in Britain

Pethidine

This analgesic and antispasmodic drug is usually given intramuscularly (50-150 mg). It is decreasing in popularity as nausea, drowsiness, and lack of control are important adverse effects.

Pethidine is considered a better analgesic by professionals than by women themselves. It works when given intramuscularly in about 20 minutes, giving good pain relief for some and

Causes of labour pain

- Stretch of the cervix during dilatation
- Ischaemia of the muscle wall of the uterus with build up of lactate
- Stretch of the vagina and perineum in the second stage

Percentages of women using pain relief (based on the reports of the National Birthday Trust surveys)

	1946	1958	1970	1984	1990
Chloroform	17	0	0	0	0
Nitrous oxide and air	16	56	2	0	0
Nitrous oxide and oxygen	0	0	52	54	60
Trilene	0	25	7	0	0
Pethidine	0	56	69	36	37
Epidural or spinal	0	3	9	17	18
Non-drug pain relief	0	1	2	13	58
No pain relief	68	34	2	2	NR

Many women used two methods and so the data are not cumulative.
NR = not recorded

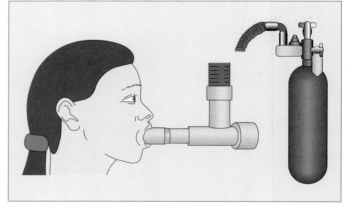

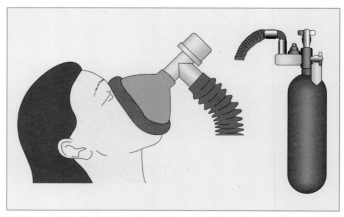

Equipment for self administration of nitrous oxide and oxygen (Entonox) with a mouth piece (top) and a face mask (bottom)

sedation for most. Because a fifth of women are nauseous with pethidine, an antiemetic—for example, metoclopramide 10 mg—is commonly given at the same time.

Pethidine crosses the placenta and is a neonatal respiratory depressant. It should be avoided in the last two hours of labour, but this is sometimes hard to judge. Naloxone reverses its effect, and the subject is considered in a later article in this series.

Morphia and diamorphine

Opiates are still used for pain relief in labour in about 5% of women in Britain, usually if epidural analgesia is not available; some 85% of women experience good pain relief with them, but they have depressive effects on neonatal respiration. In addition, morphine is frequently used after a caesarean section, via patient controlled pumps.

Epidural analgesia

Epidural analgesia provides the most effective pain relief. An indwelling plastic catheter is introduced into the epidural space through a needle with a curved tip. After the initial dose, analgesia can be extended with intermittent top ups by midwives or increasingly by the patient herself. Epidural analgesia can be given by continuous infusion via a syringe pump. It is used by about a fifth of women in England and Wales.

Traditionally, analgesia is produced with a local anaesthetic agent such as bupivacaine. This may cause motor blockade, which can be distressing. By reducing the concentration of local anaesthetic and adding an opiate such as fentanyl, good pain relief can be given in many cases with sparing of motor function. This technique is called a mobile epidural. It is not yet available in all centres.

An epidural service requires full cardiorespiratory resuscitation facilities and resident anaesthetic staff and so may not be available in small hospitals. Epidural analgesia has a very high acceptance rate: in the National Birthday Trust's latest survey over 90% of women found it to be good or very good and 85% would choose it again.

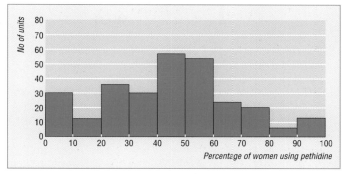

Percentage of women using pethidine by distribution of numbers of labour units in Britain

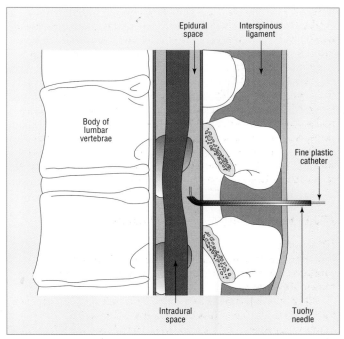

Siting of an epidural block

Mobile epidurals

- Analgesia with bupivacaine affects motor function, leading to weakness of the lower limbs
- Decreasing the concentration and adding an opiate provides good pain relief with sparing of motor function
- Ambulatory epidural service is not yet available in all centres

---

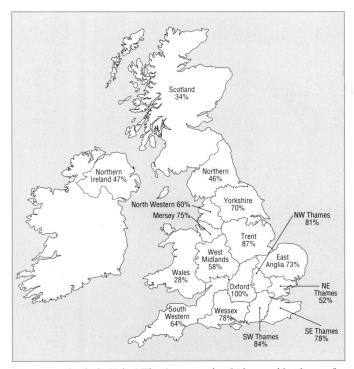

Percentage of units in United Kingdom reporting 24 hour epidural cover for labour, 1994

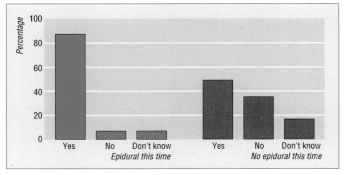

Percentage of women wishing to use epidural at next delivery

Epidurals have some potential disadvantages. The dura may be accidentally punctured; this happens in less than 1% of cases, but causes a severe postural headache in about 80% of these. This can be cured in most cases with an autologous epidural blood patch; the blood clots in the epidural space and presumably works by sealing the leak of cerebrospinal fluid, thus restoring intracranial pressure. Anyone with a severe case of headache after epidural should always be referred to the anaesthetist.

There is debate about backache after epidurals. Backache mostly occurs in patients with pre-existing problems that are exacerbated by pregnancy. Nevertheless, women should be warned of the possibility of back pain so that strain on the back can be avoided by careful positioning during the epidural.

Spinal anaesthesia

Spinal anaesthesia is increasingly used for operative procedures: caesarean section, instrumental delivery, and manual removal of the placenta. The local anaesthetic is injected into the cerebrospinal fluid through a very fine (25G) atraumatic needle. The onset of action is rapid, and the effect lasts for about two hours. Headache after a spinal injection is rare nowadays.

Nerve blocks

A pudendal nerve block with lignocaine plus an infiltration of the perineum with local anaesthetic gives good pain relief for low cavity, forceps, or vacuum extraction, but it would be unkind to use Keilland's forceps, which should be reserved for use with an epidural or spinal block. Local nerve block is an easy technique; is performed by the obstetrician at the time of delivery, and has few complications. Repair of an episiotomy is readily done under this type of analgesia.

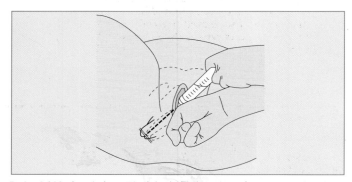

Pudendal block technique. The injection is into the pudendal nerve in the region of the ischial spine each side. The nerve usually leaves and re-enters the pelvis around this spine, but because this is not constant, anaesthesia should be located around the spine

General anaesthesia

In Britain general anaesthesia is still used for some caesarean sections, about 30% of elective procedures, and 40% of emergency procedures. It is also used for manual removal of the placenta, especially when major blood loss is anticipated.

Although general anaesthesia is relatively safe, regional anaesthesia is about eight times safer as the risks of inhaling gastric contents and of airway problems are avoided. General anaesthesia in labour is therefore decreasing.

Non-pharmacological methods

Anything that helps a woman's pain is acceptable if it does no harm. Increasing numbers of women use non-drug centred methods, possibly to maintain control, a matter of great importance to some. The least formal of these methods is the removal of anxiety—through educating the woman and a trusted companion who will be present at the birth.

> **Rates of instrumental delivery may be higher among women using an epidural because in the more painful prolonged labours with malpositions women are more likely to receive epidural analgesia**

> **Urinary retention after an epidural is best prevented by careful attention to bladder emptying**

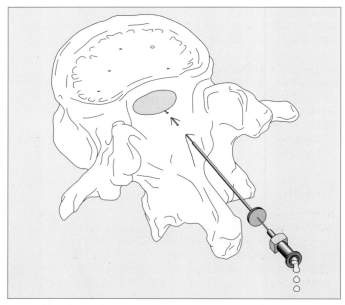

Siting of spinal anaesthetic with specially pointed atraumatic needle

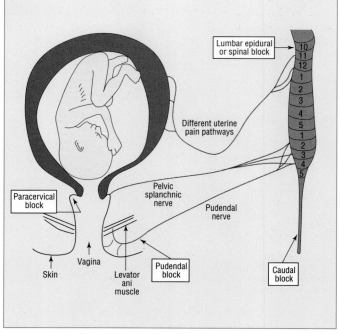

Differentiation of regional blocks (usually done by anaesthetist) and field blocks (commonly performed by obstetrician)

Relaxation and massage

Relaxation and massage are usually taught in antenatal classes. Some 90% of women find relaxation and massage to be good for pain relief. Its effectiveness depends very much on the compliance of the woman, the stage of labour at which it is used, and the availability of the partner to help.

TENS

Transcutaneous electrical nerve stimulation (TENS) is a popular method of distraction therapy. Low grade stimulatory electrical waves act on the posterior roots of the nerves supplying the uterus. TENS may postpone the need for pharmacological analgesia.

According to the National Birthday Trust's latest survey, only about 5.5% of women use TENS. A quarter of these women thought that it gave very good pain relief, but another quarter did not find it helpful. Other surveys have confirmed that it often provides only limited benefit. Machines are not usually available in NHS hospitals and have to be hired by the mother.

Warm water baths

Although the professionals may be divided about underwater births, they approve if women in labour like to use warm water baths in the first and early second stages of labour. The heat is analgesic and the buoyancy of water is relaxing. Warm water baths seem to be a good method of pain relief, although few reliable trials have been performed.

Coping with pain

In the National Birthday Trust's survey, mothers, partners, and midwives all assessed relaxation and massage as giving good or very good pain relief in almost 90% of cases. They agreed that Entonox and epidural were good in about 90% and 97% of cases respectively, but pethidine was useful in only 58% of cases.

Many women find it unhelpful to be confined to bed during labour or to have to use unwanted positions. Women usually find the presence of a companion and an individual midwife helpful in the relief of pain.

Women are often dissatisfied when they have to use a formal method of analgesia which they had initially not wished to use. This is a difficult area, which should be discussed well before labour. Women should not feel guilty about changing their mind about pain relief.

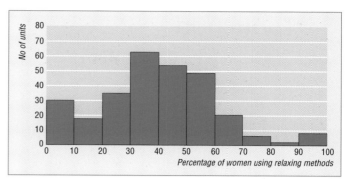

Percentage of women using relaxation methods by distribution of numbers of labour units in Britain

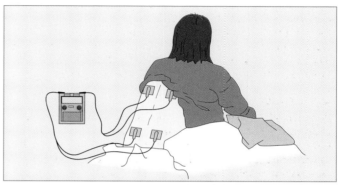

Transcutaneous electrical nerve stimulation equipment

> **Suitable pain relief in labour is difficult to predict; a woman's wishes should be assessed to see if such methods are available in the unit where she plans to deliver**

Ideal pain relief*

Should:
- Provide good analgesia
- Be safe for the mother and baby
- Be predictable and constant in its effects
- Be reversible if necessary
- Be easy to administer
- Be under the control of the mother

Should not:
- Interfere with uterine contractions
- Interfere with mobility

*A method that fulfils all of these criteria does not yet exist

Key references

- Chamberlain G, Wraight A, Steer P. *Pain and its relief in labour.* London: Parthenon Press, 1997.
- Russell R, Dundas R, Reynolds R. Long term backache after childbirth. *BMJ* 1996;312:1384-8.
- Reynolds F. Analgesia for labour. *Prescribers Journal* 1998;38:26-31.
- Leaflets on epidural pain relief are available from the Midwives' Information and Resource Unit, PO Box 669, Bristol BS99 5FG.

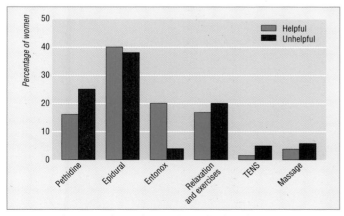

Percentage of women using various methods of pain relief and whether they found them helpful

All the graphs are adapted with permission from *Pain Relief in Labour*, the report by the National Birthday Trust.

5 Induction

Geoffrey Chamberlain, Luke Zander

Labour is induced when an external agent is used to stimulate delivery before the onset of spontaneous labour. Induction must be distinguished clearly from augmentation of labour: both use similar techniques, but the first aims to start labour, whereas the second enhances uterine contractions once labour has started.

> Induction is the stimulation of the uterus with the aim of starting labour to ensure delivery of the fetus at an appropriate time when the baby is thought to be safer outside the uterus than in it

Incidence

No statutory national data are collected on the incidence of induction. The National Birthday Trust's study on home births in 1994 showed a 19% induction rate among a normal group of women who planned to deliver in hospital compared with 0.2% in those who delivered at home. Hospital reports, where published, vary from 0% to 32%.

Induction and augmentation
- Induction means starting labour
- Augmentation means enhancing a labour that has already started

---

Indications

There are few absolute indications for inducing labour, and priorities vary with the obstetrician. Postmaturity (when the pregnancy extends well beyond the expected delivery date) still heads the list, followed by suspected fetal growth retardation and maternal hypertension. Social factors—such as the woman's own wishes—play a larger part these days.

In a meta-analysis of 10 randomised controlled trials comparing induction at 41-42 weeks with conservative treatment, Crowley showed the increased risk of perinatal deaths associated with prolonged pregnancy. The risk is reduced by induction at 41 weeks (Cochrane Collaboration).

A non-medical indication for induction is the woman's own wishes. Many mothers exceeding their expected delivery date by a week consider that their pregnancy has gone far enough and ask for induction. Roberts and Young found that about 70% of women expressed the wish to be induced after 41 weeks. Provided that the cervix is ripe, many obstetricians would agree with this choice and use a non-invasive method—for example, prostaglandins.

Maternal age and poor obstetric history are relative indications, but it should be remembered that induction is intended to result in a birth. Hence, if a vaginal delivery does not follow, a caesarean section may be required. If the grounds for induction are not strong, this could lead to a caesarean section for a poor indication.

Rarely, a planned time of delivery may be needed to provide the best care for the fetus. Some cardiac abnormalities may require immediate surgery after birth. Labour should be induced at a tertiary referral centre, with the facilities for neonatal surgery ready.

Readiness for induction

Before the obstetrician decides on induction and before he or she discusses the possibility with the woman, the uterus needs to be checked as ready for labour. This is best assessed by examining the lie and position of the fetus, the volume of amniotic fluid, the tone of the uterus, and the ripeness of the

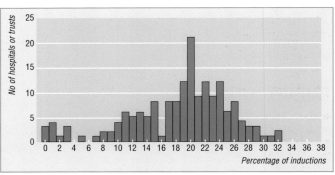

Percentage of inductions performed in hospitals or trusts in England

---

Major indications for induction of labour reported for England and Wales (1994-5) and percentage of women with such problems who were induced

	Non-cumulative % of women who were induced for this reason
Prolonged pregnancy	70
Hypertension and pre-eclampsia	51
Malposition or malpresentation of fetus	13
Pelvic abnormality	11

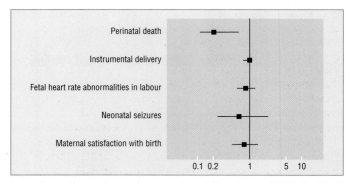

Preventing various outcomes in postpartum delivery by routine v selective induction of labour (Odds ratios of 95% Confidence Intervals)

cervix, the last being the best predictor. Some of these clinical signs have been scored by Bishop (1964), to predict cervical assessment and the likelihood of the induction being successful.

If the score exceeds 8, the chance of a successful delivery after induction is the same as that following a spontaneous onset of labour. As with many scoring systems, the Bishop's score provides only a guide. A modest correlation exists between cervical ripeness and the likelihood of success. The Bishop's score only translates into numbers what the experienced clinician learns when examining the cervix for ripeness.

When planning an induction, the obstetrician should discuss the procedure fully with the woman, explaining the method to be used, any side effects, and the sequelae if it fails. She should give her informed consent to the procedure. It may be advisable for this to be in writing; if it is not, a note should be made by the doctor in the woman's records and signed.

Contraindications

Contraindications to induction are the same as contraindications to a vaginal delivery. A few are absolute (a severe degree of placenta praevia or a transverse fetal lie); others are relative, such as active primary genital herpes infection, or a high and floating fetal head as cord prolapse could follow.

Contraindications to induction

- Severe cephalopelvic disproportion
- Severe degree of placenta praevia
- Oblique or transverse lie
- Cervix < 4 on the Bishop's score*

*This contraindication may be overcome by ripening the cervix with prostaglandins and then proceeding to induction

---

Methods of induction

Fetal maturity should first be assessed. The presentation and position of the fetus should be rechecked just before induction.

The simplest procedure is to sweep the membranes with a gloved finger lubricated with antiseptic cream and inserted gently up the cervical canal. If performed by an experienced doctor or midwife, this need not be uncomfortable. After 40 weeks' gestation, this procedure can halve the subsequent need for further induction, but at 38-40 weeks it does not significantly increase the proportion of women who go into labour within 7 days.

The traditional method of induction is to rupture the membranes, releasing amniotic fluid. The forewaters can be snagged with a simple Amnihook (EMS Medical Group), a pair of special amniotomy forceps, or a pair of Kocher's forceps. Under sterile conditions the chosen instrument is passed through the cervical canal. Under vision or digital pilotage, the forewaters are snagged. The colour of the amniotic fluid and the volume released should be assessed. The fetal heart rate should be checked immediately afterwards to ensure no fetal compromise, but it is unnecessary to continue with cardiotocography unless there is a specific indication.

Puncture of the hindwaters used to be done with a Drew Smythe catheter, an S shaped metal catheter. Although not often performed in Britain these days, this procedure is still useful in many parts of the world where access to caesarean section may be difficult. It is used for inducing a woman with an

---

Ripeness of cervix

A ripe cervix shows that a uterus is ready for labour when it is:
- Soft
- Taken up
- Dilated
- Central on the presenting part

Bishop's score used to assess cervical ripeness

Ripeness	0	1	2	3
Cervical length (cm)	>2	1 or 2	<1	Fully taken up
Cervical dilatation (cm)	0	1 or 2	3 or 4	≥5
Cervical consistency	Firm	Medium	Soft	NA
Position of cervix	Posterior	Central	Anterior	NA
Station of presenting part (cm above ischial spines)	3	2	1 or 0	Below ischial spines

---

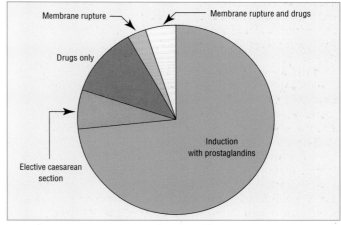

Methods of induction used in England and Wales in 1994-5

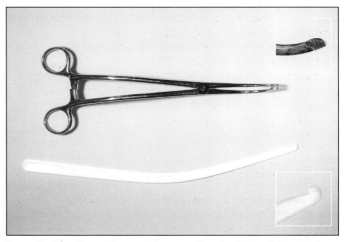

Top: pair of amniotomy forceps. Bottom: an Amnihook—plastic disposable hooked instrument

unstable lie when the fetal head is wandering out of the pelvis and needs to be stabilised.

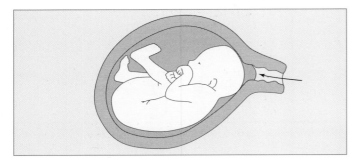

Artificial rupture of membranes by snagging at forewaters

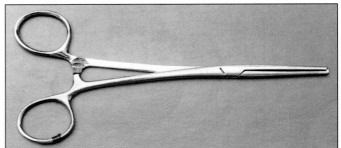

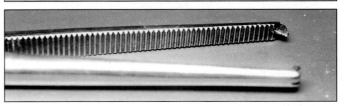

Pair of Kocher's forceps—with toothed jaws at end

Prostaglandins

The commonest method of induction in current use in the United Kingdom is with prostaglandin gel or pessaries placed high in the vagina. These hormones are the same as those produced by the uterus in early labour, so it is a more natural method than using oxytocic agents. Also, cells that have been primed with prostaglandin gel are more likely to respond if intravenous oxytocin is needed.

Prostaglandins can be given intravenously, intramuscularly, orally, or vaginally, but the first three routes often produce severe side effects and are best avoided in labour. Currently, in Britain, 1 mg or 2 mg of prostaglandin E_{2a} is given in a gel. It is absorbed into the circulation through the vaginal and cervical epithelium, returning in the blood supply to the uterus. An obstetrician or midwife starting an induction with prostaglandin gel should stay with the woman for 20-30 minutes in case of a myometrial over-reaction, and cardiotocography monitoring of the fetus is wise.

If labour is not established and the cervix is not dilating after four to six hours, the same dose of prostaglandin gel may be repeated. After this, most obstetricians would advise a low rupture of the membranes if the cervix was sufficiently ripened, usually with Syntocinon intravenously. Such a mixture should be handled with care, with a midwife constantly in attendance to observe the strength of the uterine contractions.

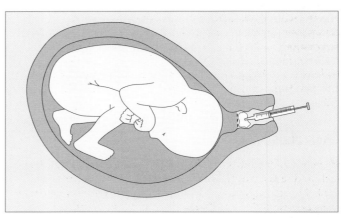

Inserting prostaglandin gel into upper vagina

Syntocinon

This synthetically produced oxytocic is given intravenously, with the dose titred against the myometrial response. For safety reasons either a very dilute solution is used or a mechanical pump is preset to inject small amounts of the concentrated agent into a dextrose saline drip. Rarely is Syntocinon used alone to induce labour; its help is more to augment existing labour after the artificial rupture of the membranes or stimulation with prostaglandin gel.

Success of induction

Insertion of prostaglandin gel into the vagina is probably the most successful method of induction overall, effective in over 90% of women. A combination of artificial rupture of the membranes and Syntocinon succeeds in 95% of women who are induced with a ripe cervix.

Failure to induce labour after correct administration of adequate doses should make the obstetrician rethink whether induction is really appropriate. If delivery is still indicated, should a caesarean section be performed? If the indications are borderline, is it possible to postpone induction for a day or so?

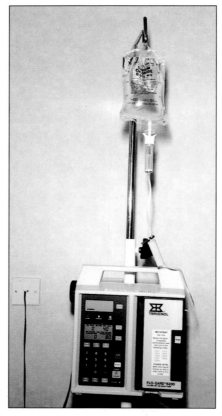

Micropump for pumping safe amounts of oxyctocic drugs into intravenous line

This can most readily be done if the membranes have not been ruptured. Such action may cause psychological reactions and the woman needs careful counselling.

Risks of induction

Induction may fail and lead to the need for caesarean section.

Uterine hyperstimulation can follow induction with Syntocinon or prostaglandin gel and lead to fetal distress, causing hypoxic damage to the baby.

Multiparous women should be induced carefully as they have an increased risk of uterine rupture. Overstimulation can be treated with tocolytics and, if the problem persists, immediate operative delivery.

Prolonged membrane rupture without delivery can result in intrauterine infection. This is less likely if labour follows within 12 hours.

If the presenting part is not well engaged, a prolapsed cord may occur with the first rush of amniotic fluid.

The risk of amniotic fluid embolism is increased.

Rarely, induction might precipitate delivery of an unexpectedly preterm infant. With ultrasound scanning in early pregnancy, this is rare.

After induction the risk of operative vaginal delivery is increased 1.5-fold and that of caesarean section is increased 1.8-fold. These may well be due to the conditions indicating induction.

Conclusions

Induction of labour is a powerful tool in obstetric management. It should be used only when the benefits to fetus or mother of the baby outweigh those of the pregnancy continuing. When induction is used, there should be sound indications and a reasonable chance that it will succeed. Using prostaglandins on their own is probably the most useful overall method.

The second graph on the first page is adapted from Crowley (*Cochrame Library*, 1998). The pie chart is adapted from the *Statistical Bulletin: NHS Maternity Statistics* (Department of Health, 1997).

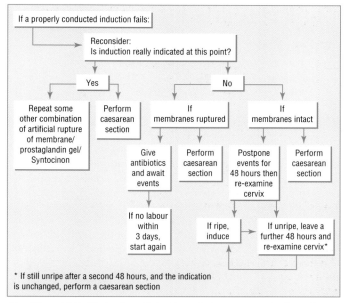

Algorithm of failed induction; all decisions depend on need for induction

Key references

- Allot H, Palmer C. Sweeping the membranes. *Br J Obstet Gynaecol* 1993;100:898-903.
- Bishop EH. Pelvic scoring for elective induction. *Obstet Gynaecol* 1964;24:267.
- Chamberlain G, Wraight A, Crowley P. *Homebirths.* Carnford: Parthenon Press, 1997:45.
- Managing post term pregnancy. *Drug and Therapeutics Bulletin* 1997;35:17-8.
- Department of Health. *Report of confidential enquiry into maternal deaths 1991-1993.* London: HMSO, 1996.
- Crowley P. Intervention to improve outcome from delivery beyond term. Elective induction of labour at 41 + weeks' gestation. In: Cochrane Collaboration. *Crochrane Library.* Issue 2. Oxford: Update Software, 1998.
- Roberts L, Young K. Management of prolonged pregnancy—women's attitudes. *Br J Obstet Gynaecol* 1991;98:1102-6.
- O'Connor R. Induction of labour—not how but why. *Br J Hosp Med* 1994;52:559-62.
- Reichler A, Romem Y, Divon MY. Induction of labor. *Curr Opin Obstet Gynecol* 1995;7:432-6.

6 Preterm labour and premature rupture of membranes

Philip Steer, Caroline Flint

The length of human pregnancy is variable; this reflects the advantages to the fetus, which would benefit by staying in the uterus to grow more, and to the mother, for whom earlier delivery might reduce pelvic damage (see the second article in the series). The result of this interaction is a relatively high incidence of premature deliveries. In the United Kingdom the incidence of preterm delivery (before 37 weeks) is about 7%, and in many developing countries, it is much higher. The baby is delivered before its homoeostatic mechanisms are properly developed and so is prone principally to the respiratory distress syndrome, hypothermia, hypoglycaemia, and jaundice.

Causes

Socioeconomic factors influence the incidence of preterm labour. Preterm birth is significantly more common in young women, those with low body weight (body mass index < 19), those of lower social class, unmarried or unsupported mothers, and smokers. Some medical factors may increase the risk of preterm birth—for example, previous preterm delivery, persistent vaginal bleeding in early pregnancy, and heart disease. Cervical incompetence is a rare cause of preterm labour, sometimes preventable by cervical cerclage (a purse string suture around the cervix as close to the internal os as possible). The Medical Research Council's trial showed a small but significant benefit from this procedure, even in women with equivocal risk factors.

Risk factors for preterm labour

- Young age of mother (≤15 years)
- Lower socioeconomic class
- Unmarried or unsupported
- Underweight
- Cigarette smoking
- Previous preterm baby
- Multiple pregnancy
- Cervical incompetence
- Premature rupture of the membranes

Infection, usually chorioamnionitis, is a significant component in many cases of spontaneous preterm labour. The ascent of any organism through the cervical mucus plug into the uterus stimulates an inflammatory reaction in the placenta, fetal membranes, and maternal decidua. This leads to the release of cytokines such as interleukin 1β and interleukin 6 from endothelial cells and tumour necrosis α from macrophages. These stimulate the cascade of prostaglandin production, which in turn produces cervical ripening and uterine contractions. The commonest groups of organisms are the streptococci, mycoplasmas, and fusiform bacilli. Bacterial vaginosis (*Gardnerella vaginalis*) associated with a vaginal pH value of 5.4 seems to promote preterm labour, possibly reducing the efficiency of the cervical barrier to infection. Preliminary studies suggest that treatment with metronidazole or clindamycin in women with bacterial vaginosis may reduce the incidence of preterm labour, and prospective studies are under way.

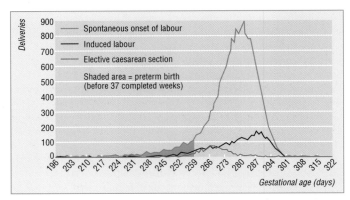

Distribution of 24 675 deliveries by gestational age (determined by early ultrasound scanning dates) for a British maternity hospital (Queen's Medical Centre, Nottingham), 1988-95

Major risks of early preterm delivery

- Death
- Respiratory distress syndrome
- Hypothermia
- Hypoglycaemia
- Necrotising enterocolitis
- Jaundice
- Infection
- Retinopathy of prematurity

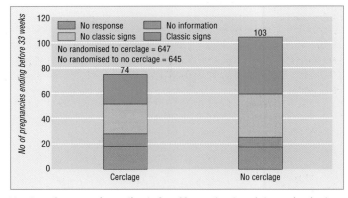

Number of pregnancies ending before 33 completed weeks' gestation in the Medical Research Council and Royal College of Obstetricians and Gynaecologists' cervical cerclage trial, classified by whether they had signs typical of cervical incompetence (painless cervical dilatation and rupture of the membranes before 30 weeks' gestation)

Major causes of preterm labour

- Iatrogenic (induction for medical reasons)
- Infection
- Premature rupture of the membranes
- Multiple pregnancy
- Polyhydramnios
- Intrauterine death
- Fetal abnormalities
- Uterine abnormalities
- Cervical incompetence

About 30% of preterm births are iatrogenic—that is, induced by obstetricians for maternal indications such as fulminating pre-eclampsia or for fetal indications such as severe intrauterine growth restriction. In recent years, since the increased use of assisted reproduction, multiple pregnancy has become a growing cause of preterm labour. The incidence of fetal abnormality is higher in pregnancies complicated by preterm labour.

Diagnosis of preterm labour

The precise diagnosis of preterm labour is not easy. The only absolute proof is progressive dilatation of the cervix, but once this has happened, it is too late to attempt preventive treatment. The finding of fetal fibronectin, a fetal protein involved in cell to cell adhesion, in vaginal secretions suggests that the cervical mucus plug is becoming ineffective. This has been proposed as a sensitive screen for preterm labour, but its poor specificity, together with a relatively high false positive rate, makes it unsuitable for routine use.

The diagnosis of labour often has to be made on the basis of reported uterine contractions. However, Braxton Hicks contractions are noticed in most pregnancies from about 24 weeks' gestation onwards, and many women find these painful. This means that the diagnosis of preterm labour is often wrong; two thirds of women diagnosed as being in labour will not have delivered within 48 hours, and over one third go to term. Diagnosis with home uterine contraction monitoring has been tested in a number of trials, but no consensus on its value has emerged.

Diagnosis remains essentially clinical, with a careful history and a speculum examination being important components. Abdominal pain of any type, or any vaginal bleeding, requires a careful speculum examination of the cervix. Digital examinations should be avoided if there is any suggestion of ruptured membranes as they increase the risk of ascending infection. Seeing amniotic fluid trickling through the cervix remains the only certain way of diagnosing ruptured membranes. The use of an acidity indicator, such as nitrazine sticks (Amnicator, Corsham), is not reliable, as this indicates only that the vagina is no longer acid, an effect that can be produced by urine or bath water.

When examining the cervix, a vaginal swab should be taken for culture. This will enable appropriate antibiotic treatment if signs of infection develop later.

Management

Tocolysis

Suppression of uterine contractions would seem to be the obvious solution to the problem of preterm labour. However, tocolytic agents do not work effectively for longer than about 48 hours, probably because of tachyphylaxis. Their major use is to postpone delivery—for example, for *in utero* transfer to a tertiary centre—or to allow the administration of corticosteroids to the mother and so to her fetus to promote surfactant release in the fetal lung and reduce the incidence of the neonatal respiratory distress syndrome by up to 50%. This effect is only significant at gestations up to 34 weeks; after this it is usual to allow preterm labour to progress.

However, there are many situations in which the use of tocolytics is inappropriate. In a typical maternity unit, delivering about 3000 women a year, only about 50 women a year will be suitable for tocolysis (about one a week).

Incidence of multiple pregnancy per 1000 multiple births in United Kingdom

	1985	1990	1995
All multiple pregnancies	10.4	11.6	14.1
Twins	10.2	11.3	13.6
Triplets	0.14	0.28	0.44

All multiple pregnancy births increased about 1.4-fold; triplets increased threefold.

Accuracy of fibronectin testing in prediction of preterm delivery: meta-analysis of 723 symptomatic and 847 asymptomatic women. Values are probability percentages, unless stated otherwise; values in parentheses are 95% confidence intervals

	Pretest	Post-test		Likelihood ratio %
		Positive results	Negative results	
Symptomatic women:				
Delivery <34 weeks	32.5 (24.2 to 40.8)	55.6 (43.4 to 67.3)	8.2 (8.1 to 20.1)	2.6 (1.8 to 3.7); 0.2 (0.1 to 0.5)
Delivery within 1 week of testing	6.6 (4.3 to 8.9)	25.8 (18.0 to 35.5)	1.2 (0.4 to 3.1)	5.0 (3.8 to 6.4); 0.2 (0.1 to 0.6)
Asymptomatic women:				
At high risk delivering at <34 weeks	15.7 (10.3 to 21.1)	31.0 (21.3 to 42.6)	9.9 (5.6 to 16.7)	2.4 (1.8 to 3.2); 0.6 (0.4 to 0.9)
At low risk delivering at <37 weeks	25.0 (23.4 to 39.6)	52.0 (41.2 to 62.6)	22.0 (18.8 to 25.5)	3.2 (2.2 to 4.8); 0.8 (0.7 to 0.9)

Likelihood ratio = the probability of a positive (or negative) result among women with a preterm delivery compared with the probability of such a result in those without a preterm delivery.

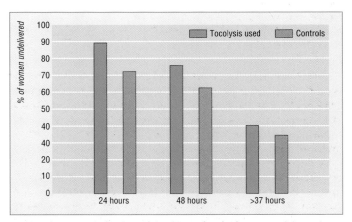

Results of meta-analysis of 16 trials of betamimetics in preterm labour. A high proportion of women remained undelivered without any treatment (therefore original diagnosis of preterm labour was erroneous)

Tocolytics are only of value in about an eighth of preterm labours

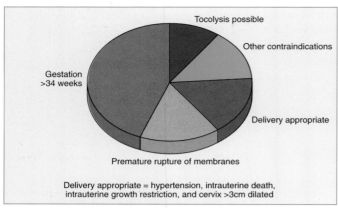

Delivery appropriate = hypertension, intrauterine death, intrauterine growth restriction, and cervix >3cm dilated

Possible use of tocolysis in 1445 preterm labours

Many tocolytics are currently used. Sympathomimetics such as ritodrine and salbutamol are generally the safest choice for the mother and fetus, although they can cause tachycardia and pulmonary oedema if given in overdose. Indomethacin can be used before 32 weeks, and because it restricts fetal urine output it is useful if there is polyhydramnios. However, it may cause premature closure of the fetal ductus arteriosus if used after 32 weeks' gestation, which can lead to significant pulmonary hypertension. Alcohol and isoxuprine hydrochloride are no longer used, while calcium channel blockers cause significant hypotension. Atosiban, an oxytocin antagonist, shows promise, as does nimesulide, a selective cyclo-oxygenase type 2 inhibitor. Nitric oxide donors such as glyceryl trinitrate are also being evaluated. No evidence exists that prophylactic tocolytics, given orally throughout the first and second trimesters of pregnancy, are of benefit.

When the membranes have ruptured, the use of tocolytics is controversial. The concern is that contractions may result from occult chorioamnionitis, and suppressing labour could allow infection to spread. If tocolytics are used in this situation—for example, to allow transfer of the baby *in utero* to a tertiary centre—intravenous broad spectrum antibiotics should probably also be given. The routine administration of antibiotics with ruptured membranes has not been proved to be valuable and is currently the subject of the ORACLE trial. Most cases will be managed conservatively, with labour being induced at 36 weeks. Close observation for signs of a developing infection is mandatory; monitoring of maternal temperature, white blood cell count, and blood concentrations of C reactive protein is usual. In the United States amniocentesis is sometimes used to screen for occult infection but has not been shown to be effective in prospective trials and is rarely performed in Britain. Re-examinations of the vagina should be avoided, as they increase the risk of infection.

Antenatal steroids

Meta-analyses of the use of tocolytics suggest that they have little effect on perinatal mortality. However, they do allow time for the administration of antenatal steroids, which, if given at least 24-48 hours before birth, can halve the incidence and severity of respiratory distress and mortality in newborn infants. The effect of steroids lasts up to about a week. The benefit of repeated doses of steroids to the fetus has not been shown; their safety and efficacy needs to be tested in a prospective trial.

Preterm delivery

The preferred method of delivery in preterm labour depends on the fetal presentation and the stage of gestation. If the baby is presenting by the head, then vaginal delivery is probably safe

Tocolytics

Currently used
- β sympathomimetics, such as ritodrine, terbutaline, salbutamol
- Magnesium sulphate (used particularly in the United States)
- Prostaglandin synthase inhibitors, such as unselective (indomethacin) and selective (cyclo-oxygenase type 2—nimesulide)
- Nitric oxide donors, such as glyceryl trinitrate
- Calcium channel blockers, such as nifedipine

No longer used
- Alcohol
- Isoxuprine

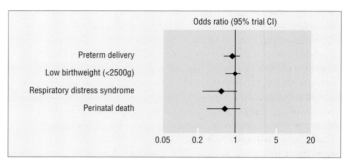

Results of meta-analysis of prophylactic action of betamimetics in pregnancy—effect on selected outcomes in 11 trials

The ORACLE study
- This multicentre study is investigating the usefulness of antibiotics when membranes rupture prematurely—particularly, whether they reduce the risk of early preterm labour and improve the baby's chances of survival
- The antibiotics being used in the study are Augmentin and erythromycin
- Women take the antibiotics (or placebo) for 10 days or until the birth of their baby, whichever is the shorter time

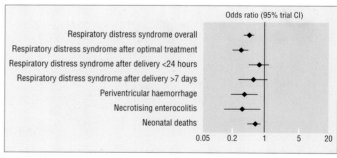

Results of meta-analysis of effect of corticosteroids before delivery in selected outcomes in 15 trials

Potential neonatal hazards of repeated antenatal steroids

Animal studies	*Human studies*
Growth delay	Sepsis
Neurodevelopmental delay	Necrotising enterocolitis
Induced hypertension	Reduced head
Long term breathing problems	circumference
Adrenal suppression	

in most cases, with caesarean delivery being performed only for the usual obstetric indications. In a breech presentation before 32 weeks it is possibly safer for the baby to be delivered by cesarean section. This, however, considerably raises the risk to the mother as in many cases the operation is not straightforward because the lower segment may not be well formed.

The preterm baby

The conditions into which the baby is born have a major influence on its chance of survival. Very preterm babies (those born at less than 28 weeks) do best when delivered in a tertiary referral centre with a neonatal intensive care unit. Deliveries should be conducted by experienced midwives or obstetricians, with an experienced paediatrician present. The delivery room should be warm, and there should be adequate equipment for resuscitation (see final article in this series). If preterm labour starts at home, or in a smaller hospital, transfer of the mother in early labour should be considered, for the mother is the ideal incubator. However, in some cases the mother is also unwell—for example, with high blood pressure—and her condition must be taken into account. In one study 17% of such mothers ended their transfer in the adult intensive care unit. Care must be taken to stabilise maternal condition before transfer. Transfer is probably unwise if labour is progressing rapidly or there is substantial vaginal bleeding.

Modern neonatal intensive care means that babies delivered after 30 weeks' gestation usually survive intact. However, babies delivered between 23 and 24 weeks' gestation have an increased risk of long term handicap. With babies at the limit of viability (23-24 weeks), both a paediatrician and an obstetrician should, whenever possible, discuss management with the parents, as the likelihood of handicap may exceed 50%.

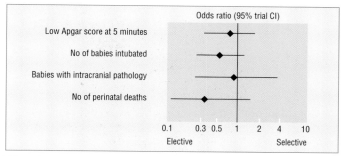

Effect of elective *v* selective caesarean delivery for preterm breech births

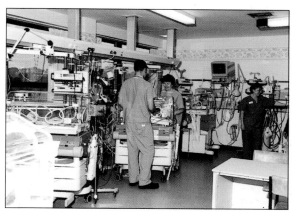

Neonatal intensive care unit

Conclusion

- Preterm labour needs careful management in centres with staff skilled in this field
- Antenatal steroids are of significant benefit and should always be given
- Discussion about prognosis and plans for delivery must include the paediatricians

Key references

- Morrison J, Rennie J. Aspects of fetal and neonatal care at extreme preterm periods of gestation. *Br J Obstet Gynaecol* 1997;104:1341-50.
- Royal College of Obstetricians and Gynaecologists. *Beta agonists for the care of women in preterm labour.* London: RCOG, 1997. (Guideline No 1A.)
- Royal College of Obstetricians and Gynaecologists. *Antenatal corticosteroids to prevent RDS.* London: RCOG, 1996. (Guideline No 7.)

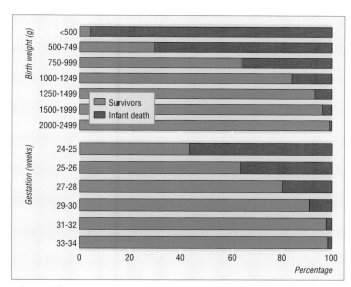

Infant survival to 1 year in Wales, by birth weight and gestation—cumulative data 1993-5

The box listing potential neonatal hazards of antenatal steroids is based on an article by Quinlivan et al (*Aust NZ J Obstet Gynaecol* 1998;38:1-7). The table on fibronectin testing is adapted from Chien P et al (*Br J Obstet Gynaecol* 1997;104:436-44). The graph of distribution of deliveries by gestational age is adapted from Gardosi et al (*Br J Obstet Gynaecol* 1997;104:792-7). The histogram from the cerclage trial is adapted from the MRC/RCOG Working Party (*Br J Obstet Gynaecol* 1993;100:516-23). The chart showing use of tocolysis is adapted from Tucker et al (*Obstet Gynecol* 1991;77:343-7). The graph showing the meta-analysis of prophylactic betamimetics in pregnancy is adapted from Keirse (*Cochrane Pregnancy and Childbirth Database*; Oxford: Update Software, 1995). The graph showing the meta-analysis of effect of corticosteroids before delivery is adapted from Crowley (*Cochrane Pregnancy and Childbirth Database*; Oxford: Update Software, 1995). The graph of caesarean delivery is adapted from Grant et al (*Br J Obstet Gynaecol* 1996;103:1197-200). The bar chart showing survival rates is adapted from Emsley et al (*Arch Dis Childhood* 1998;78:F99-104). The photograph of the neonatal intensive care unit was taken by Douglas Neil, medical photographer at the Singleton Hospital.

7   Labour in special circumstances

Geoffrey Chamberlain, Philip Steer

About two thirds of labours are normal. In the rest, increased surveillance—and sometimes action—is required to prevent maternal or fetal problems. All overall care givers need to be able to recognise such variations and either take appropriate action or refer to an obstetrician for advice and assistance. This may require transfer to hospital if the woman is in labour at home or in a freestanding general practitioner unit. A paediatrician should be called to attend if any problems are anticipated.

Slow progress (delay) in labour

The fundamental process of labour is progressive dilatation of the cervix. The woman herself usually diagnoses labour when she has recurrent painful uterine contractions. However, such contractions may be ripening the cervix (the latent phase) before rapid cervical dilatation (the active phase) occurs. Midwives and doctors judge progress by assessing the descent of the fetal presenting part on abdominal palpation and advancement of the fetus on vaginal examination (position of the presenting part relative to the ischial spines). These may be imprecise measurements, but a series of careful assessments by the same observer is usually informative.

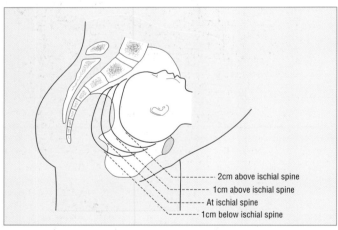

The concept of the fetal head descending through the pelvis in labour is checked by vaginal examination when the level of the presenting part is assessed against the level of the ischial spines (in centimetres) vertically

Labour is usually diagnosed by the professional when there are regular contractions or when the cervix has reached 3 cm dilatation in the presence of contractions. At this point, the recording of details on a partogram is often started. Intervention to accelerate labour in the latent phase is not associated with an improvement in outcome, but pain relief with an epidural and augmentation of labour are sometimes necessary to prevent the woman becoming exhausted and demoralised.

The woman should not be left alone in labour; usually her partner is there, and the midwife should be constantly available if not actually in the room. Adequate pain relief should be given

> **The commonest problem in childbirth is a labour that is progressing slowly**

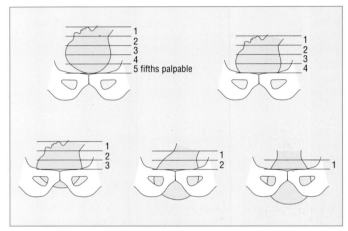

Descent of the fetal head into the pelvis is checked by abdominal examination when the head is imagined in segments of one fifth. Engagement—when the maximum diameter of the fetal head has entered the pelvis—corresponds with only two fifths of the head being palpable through the abdomen

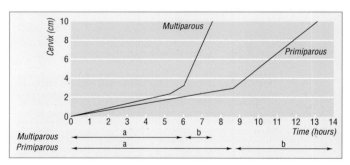

Latent (a) and active (b) phase of labour in a multiparous and a primiparous woman, as shown on partogram

---

Information conveyed on a partogram

- Fetal heart rate—by intermittent auscultation or continuous fetal heart rate monitoring
- Cervicogram—a record of cervical dilatation and fetal head descent
- Uterine contractions—quantification of frequency, strength, and duration
- Amniotic fluid (if the membranes are ruptured)—state of fluid, any meconium
- Maternal urine production—checked for ketones and protein
- Drugs given—analgesics, oxytocics
- Maternal blood pressure, pulse, and temperature

(see earlier article). It used to be recommended that women should be starved during labour, but such restrictions are now considered unnecessary if progress is normal and there is no significant risk of a caesarean section. Fluids and a light diet are allowed.

The rate of cervical dilatation in the active phase at which augmentation of labour is indicated is controversial. In the 1960s through to the early 1980s O'Driscoll and colleagues suggested that any nulliparous woman with a rate of cervical dilatation below the average (1 cm/h) should be augmented. Thus active management would be used in half of women in their first pregnancies; few multiparous women progress this slowly. Most obstetricians in Britain are now more conservative, and 0.5 cm/h is commonly taken as the cut off. Usually the first step in augmentation is to rupture the amniotic membranes; if this is not followed by a speedy labour intravenous oxytocin is given to stimulate contractions. Careful clinical monitoring is needed to ensure that contractions do not exceed one every two minutes, or fetal hypoxia may result from restriction of the maternal afferent placental blood flow.

When the progress of labour is so slow (despite oxytocic stimulation) that the woman is becoming exhausted and the fetus at risk of hypoxia, a caesarean section is the likely solution. An individual decision is taken by each woman on the recommendation of her obstetrician and often her paediatrician. A caesarean section cannot be performed without the mother's specific consent, except when she is mentally incompetent; the decision must then be made by a court.

Cephalopelvic disproportion

Disparity between the size of the fetus and the mother's pelvis is uncommon in Britain, but it is still a major problem in the developing world.

The disparity may be absolute or relative. Absolute disparity occurs when there is no possibility of vaginal delivery; in relative disparity, the baby may be large, but if the head is well flexed and uterine contractions are good, delivery can be achieved after a long, hard labour.

Some causes of absolute disproportion

- A very big baby (>5 kg birth weight)
- Fetal hydrocephalus
- Congenitally abnormal pelvis where the sacral alae are missing
- Pelvis that has been damaged by trauma
- Pelvis contracted after oesteomalacia in youth

If in late pregnancy in a nulliparous woman the fetal head is not engaged, and will not do so, suspicion should be aroused. The success of labour depends not only on pelvic size but also on the compliance of the soft tissues, the efficiency of the uterine contractions, the ability of the fetal head to mould, and the position it takes up in labour. Most women are now recommended to have a trial of labour unless they have major pelvic problems. If imaging before labour is necessary, computed tomography exposes the fetus to fewer x rays than do plain films (and magnetic resonance imaging to none) and is more accurate.

The phrase "trial of labour" is awesome but does warn the labour ward staff that cephalopelvic disproportion is suspected. Oxytocin should be used with caution, to avoid overstimulation of the uterus. A partogram is particularly valuable, and if the woman's progress lies to the right of the expected curve, a

---

> Labour progress is different in primiparous and multiparous women and is best displayed graphically on a partogram, which shows average dilatation rates by parity

---

Percentages of women receiving active management of labour, promoted by O'Driscoll and colleagues in the 1960s, '70s, and '80s

	1968	1972	1980
Augmentation	11	55	41
Caesarean section in labour	1.2	1.8	1.2

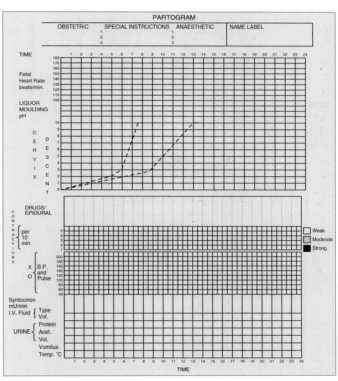

Partogram: the broken lines show expected progress of cervical dilatation in multiparous (left) and primiparous (right) women

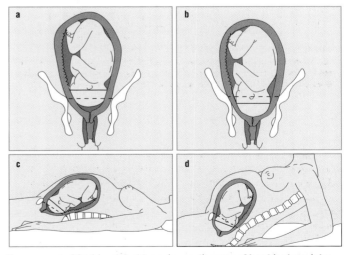

Engagement of fetal head. In (a) maximum diameter of head is above inlet of pelvis and head is not engaged; in (b) engagement has taken place (maximum diameter of head is below inlet of pelvis); in (c) head is not engaged; in (d) when mother sits up on her elbows, the head sinks in, an indication that the head will engage when labour starts

caesarean section should be considered while the woman is not exhausted and the fetus is not distressed. It is important to involve the woman and her partner as fully and early as possible in any decisions obtaining relevant consent.

Fulminating pre-eclampsia and eclampsia

Hypertension induced by pregnancy (a blood pressure of ≥140/90 mm Hg on two occasions at least 6 hours apart) is quite common, with an incidence of 5-12% depending on the population. Pre-eclampsia (hypertension with proteinuria of at least 300 mg/l) is less common, occurring in only 1-2%. If pre-eclampsia progresses into eclampsia, it becomes an acute emergency.

Presenting symptoms in 442 women with fulminating pre-eclampsia

	%
Epigastric pain	65
Nausea and vomiting	36
Headache (mainly frontal)	31
Visual field disturbances	10
Bleeding	9
Jaundice	5

Symptoms of severe pre-eclampsia include acute headache, visual disturbances, vomiting with upper abdominal pain as the liver peritoneum is stretched by oedema, or subcapsular haemorrhage. On examination, reflexes will be very brisk, even to the state of clonus; blood pressure may have risen even higher, and there will be increased proteinuria. In severe cases the HELLP (Haemolysis, Elevated Liver enzymes, and Low Platelets) syndrome may develop.

Currently, the drug of choice is magnesium sulphate, given by intravenous infusion. It substantially reduces the risk of fitting, reduces blood pressure, and relaxes the uterus. Hydralazine is sometimes needed to reduce the arterial blood pressure further if the magnesium sulphate alone is not sufficient, but it is not necessary to reduce the blood pressure below 140/90 mm Hg; indeed, doing so may compromise placental perfusion.

Women with cardiac disease

Rheumatic fever as a cause of heart valve damage has greatly decreased in Britain over the past 50 years because of better housing and the use of antibiotics. As a result of the developments in cardiac surgery in the 1960s and '70s, many women with congenital heart disease now survive to childbearing age (about 0.5% of all women booking).

Despite a common belief that caesarean section is an easy option in such cases, a straightforward spontaneous labour with epidural analgesia to mitigate stress, and a well assisted second stage, is associated with the lowest morbidity and mortality. The priority in management is to prevent complications such as prolonged labour and infection, while being careful not to introduce destabilising iatrogenic factors such as epidural hypotension and fluid overload.

Detailed surveillance with intra-arterial blood pressure measurement, maternal electrocardiographic monitoring, and pulse oximetry is important.

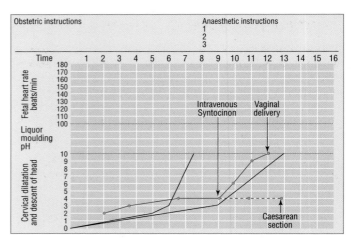

Delay in first stage of labour in a multiparous woman. The line of cervical dilatation is flattened and crosses the expected line, leading to a change of management to increase uterine contractions. If this works, progress speeds up and runs in parallel to the expected line, leading to a vaginal delivery. If it does not, a caesarean section should follow after a reasonable trial—in this case, 4 hours

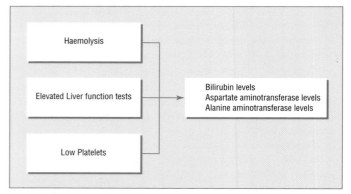

Biological and haematological symptoms of HELLP (Haemolysis, Elevated Liver enzymes, Low Platelets) syndrome

Emergency intravenous drug regimens for eclampsia

- Magnesium sulphate
- Diazepam
- Hydralazine
- Labetalol
- Phenytoin

Senior, experienced medical and obstetric staff should be involved at all times in the labour of women with cardiac disease

Women with HIV infection

Women known to be HIV positive should be taking zidovudine and protease inhibitors during the second half of pregnancy. This reduces the viral load in the blood and therefore reduces the risk of infecting the baby at birth (by about 50%).

To reduce this risk even further, an intravenous infusion of zidovudine for 4 hours is recommended just before anticipated delivery. Elective caesarean section has been shown to reduce the risk even further (by another 40%). The lower uterine segment incision should be made using a staple gun to seal the wound edges, thus ensuring an almost bloodless field through which the baby can be delivered.

If the mother chooses a vaginal birth, the application of scalp electrodes and fetal blood sampling breach the baby's skin and may increase the risk of infection; these procedures should therefore be avoided. Avoidance of breast feeding also halves the overall risk of infection (it carries at 15% risk).

Use of all known techniques for prophylaxis reduces the overall risk of fetal and neonatal infection from about 30% to under 5% (and possibly below 1%).

> It is important that pregnant women are screened for HIV infection; an infected woman can then be offered care to protect her baby, and staff too can be properly protected

Key references

- *Confidential enquiry into stillbirths and deaths in infancy.* London: Maternal and Child Health Research Consortium , 1998. (5th annual report.)
- Erikim M, Kievse M, Refrew M, Neilson J. *Guide to effective care in pregnancy and childbirth.* 2nd ed. Oxford: Oxford University Press, 1993:145.
- James D, Steer P, Weiner C, Gonik B. *High risk pregnancy—management options.* London: Saunders, 1999.
- Mercey D. Antenatal HIV testing. *BMJ* 1998;316:241-2.

The table showing active management of labour is based on data from O'Driscoll et al (*BMJ* 1969;ii:447-8; *BMJ* 1973;iii:135-7; and *Obstet Gynecol* 1984;63:485-90). The drawing of fetal head engagement is adapted from Chamberlain (*ABC of antenatal care.* London: BMJ Publishing, 1996).

8 Unusual presentations and positions and multiple pregnancy

Geoffrey Chamberlain, Philip Steer

In the vast majority of deliveries near term the fetus presents by the head, with the best fit into the lower pelvis in the occipito-anterior position. However, although the head is presenting, it may be not in an occipito-anterior but in an occipito-posterior or -transverse position. In a few cases the head is grossly deflexed so that the brow or even the face can present.

In other instances, it is not the head that is at the lower pole of the uterus but the buttocks, or breech (from the old English brec—breeches or buttocks). The fetus many even lie transversely so that no pole is in relation to the pelvic inlet. A fetus in this position is undeliverable vaginally; both transverse lies and breech presentations are much more common if the woman enters labour in the earlier weeks of pregnancy (22-28 weeks of gestation).

All these malpresentations and malpositions need careful diagnosis and skilful management.

Malpositions

Normal mechanism
Usually the fetal head engages in the left (less commonly, right) occipito-anterior position and then undergoes a short rotation to be directly occipito-anterior in the mid-cavity.

Occipito-posterior position
This is the commonest malpresentation. The head engages in the left or right occipito-transverse position, and the occiput rotates posteriorly, rather than into the more favourable occipito-anterior position. The reasons for the malrotation are often unclear. A flat sacrum or a head that is poorly flexed may be responsible; alternatively, poor uterine contractions may not push the head down into the pelvis strongly enough to produce correct rotation; epidural analgesia might sometimes relax the pelvic floor to an extent that the fetal occiput sinks into it rather than being pushed to rotate in an anterior direction. The diagnosis is determined clinically by vaginal examination.

The best management is to await events, preparing the woman and staff for a long labour. Progress should be monitored by abdominal and vaginal assessment, and the mother's condition should be watched closely. Good pain relief with an epidural and adequate hydration are required.

The mother may have an urge to push before full dilation, but the midwife should discourage this. If the occiput comes directly into the posterior position (face to pubis) a vaginal delivery is possible if the pelvic diameters are reasonable.

Occipito-transverse position
The head engages in the left or right occipito-transverse position, but then rotation to occipito-anterior fails to occur and the head remains in the transverse position. If the second stage is reached the head must be manually rotated, rotated with appropriate forceps (namely, those with no pelvic curve—for example, Kielland's forceps), or delivered using vacuum extraction.

Such vaginal deliveries must not be undertaken if there is any acidosis (fetal blood pH < 7.15) as cerebral haemorrhage may result. They are now often undertaken in the operating theatre (trial of forceps) so that a rapid change to caesarean

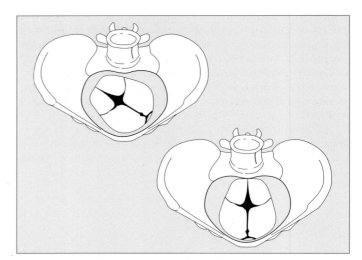

Fetal head engages in left occipito-anterior position (top) then descends into mid-cavity and rotates to full occipito-anterior (bottom)

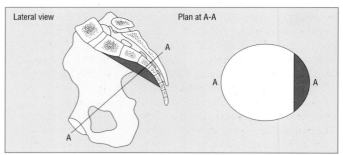

If, instead of the normal curve, the sacrum is straightened (shaded area), the anterior-posterior diameter in mid-cavity is reduced (A-A), thus hindering head rotation in this zone

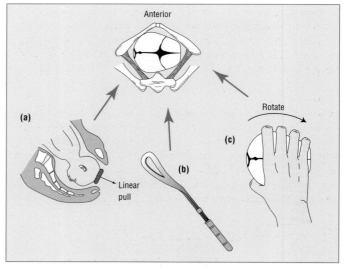

Three methods of delivering a baby in occipito-transverse position in the second stage of labour: (a) vacuum extraction with a linear pull, so allowing rotation to occur according to the pelvic anatomy; (b) rotation and extraction with Kielland's (straight) forceps; or (c) manual rotation of head and then forceps applied immediately, once occipito-anterior position is achieved

section can be made if there is any difficulty. Some obstetricians have abandoned these more difficult vaginal deliveries in favour of caesarean section.

Face and brow positions

If there is a complete extension of the fetal head, the face will present for delivery. Labour will be longer, but if the pelvis is adequate and the head rotates to a mentoanterior position, a vaginal delivery can be expected. If the head rotates backwards to a mentoposterior position a caesarean section is needed.

In a brow presentation the fetal head stays between full extension and full flexion so that the biggest diameter (the mento-vertex 13 cm) presents. This is usually only diagnosed once labour is well established. Unless the head flexes, a vaginal delivery is not possible, and a caesarean section is required.

Malpresentations

Breech

This is the commonest malpresentation. It is usually discovered before labour, although some are not diagnosed until during labour, when vaginal examinations allow a more precise diagnosis to be made, especially as the cervix dilates and allows direct palpation of the presenting part of the fetus. Current opinion holds that in late pregnancy, external cephalic version should be offered, with the use of tocolytics in nulliparous women to relax the uterus. This procedure is successful in 40% of nulliparous women, and 60% of multiparous women if performed after 38 weeks. If breech presentation persists, preparations for delivery are made. Delivery should be in a hospital with an experienced midwife and obstetrician actively involved. An anaesthetist and paediatrician should be available.

With a normal pelvis and the fetus's weight estimated by ultrasonography to be 2500-3500 g, assisted breech delivery in experienced hands is probably as safe as a caesarean section. These days many women with a breech presentation choose to have a caesarean section as they think this is the safest method of delivery. In the past doctors have led them to believe this, but meta-analyses of randomised controlled trials do not substantiate this view. Of those women who aim for a vaginal delivery, about half will succeed. Before 32 weeks, caesarean section is commonly performed for a breech presentation, although the evidence of its effectiveness even at this gestation is not strong; the operation can be technically difficult, leading to maternal complications (see next chapter).

Breech delivery is an art that all those practising obstetrics need to learn, with supervision by senior practitioners, because unexpected breech deliveries still occur.

Transverse lie

When the fetus is lying sideways with the head in one flank and the buttocks in the other, it cannot be born vaginally. Unless it converts or is converted in late pregnancy, a caesarean section is required. After opening the abdominal wall, the surgeon may be able through the wall of the uterus to rotate the fetus so that it then becomes a longitudinal lie. If not, the uterine incision must be so placed transversely to allow access to a fetal pole.

Prolapsed umbilical cord

If the presenting part of the fetus does not fit the pelvis after membrane rupture, the umbilical cord can slip past and present at the cervix, or actually prolapse into the vagina. If such an event is diagnosed in labour, the woman should be transferred straight to a hospital, preferably in a steep lateral or knee chest

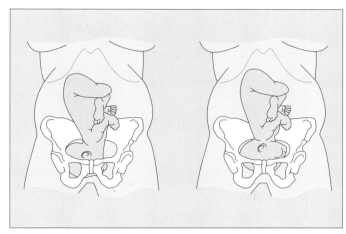

Left: Abdominal features of a face presentation; the head is felt on the same side as the back and is often not engaged. Right: Abdominal features of a brow presentation—both the sinciput and the occiput are equally palpable on each side of the lower abdomen; the head is commonly not engaged

> **All women with malpresentations and malpositions should be delivered in hospital**

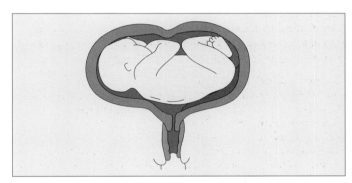

Transverse lie with subseptate uterus and low lying placenta

Vaginal delivery of breech presentation

- The mother should be in the lithotomy position (laterally tilted to avoid supine hypotension)
- The bladder should be emptied
- An anaesthetist and a paediatrician should be present
- An episiotomy is advisable
- The breech, legs, and abdomen should be allowed to deliver spontaneously (the legs can be assisted by flexing)
- The shoulders can be encouraged to deliver by rotation of the trunk. Lövsett's manoeuvre if arms extended
- Delivery of the head should be controlled manually or with forceps

> **Nowadays internal podalic version is not often attempted in transverse lies; a caesarean section is thought to be safer, although it can be a difficult operation**

position with a midwife holding up the presenting part with fingers in the vagina, to stop it compressing the umbilical cord during contractions. A caesarean section is needed urgently.

If the cord is found ahead of the presenting part before membrane rupture, the membranes should not be ruptured artificially unless full preparations for an emergency caesarean section have been made. The cord often slips up to one side of the head and disappears when the membranes rupture.

Shoulder dystocia

After delivery of the head the hardest part of delivery is usually over, but occasionally the shoulders are slightly broader than usual, with a bisacromial diameter greater than 10 cm. The shoulders usually adopt the antero-posterior axis to negotiate the outlet. If the shoulders are still above the brim at this stage, no advance occurs. The baby's chest is trapped within a vaginal cuirass. Although the nose and mouth are outside, the chest cannot expand with respiration. There is currently no way of predicting this problem reliably. The fifth annual report from the confidential inquiry into stillbirths and deaths in infancy (1998) considers the problem well. Expert help is needed.

Multiple pregnancies

Multiple pregnancies are increasing in frequency in Britain, mainly as a result of infertility treatment (both ovarian stimulation and in vitro fertilisation). Nearly all multiple pregnancies are now diagnosed early by ultrasound examination. Sometimes one twin dies and is absorbed in the first half of pregnancy (the disappearing twin syndrome). When pregnant with twins, most women go into labour early at about 37 weeks. The woman should be in labour in a hospital with a special care baby unit. With no complicating factors, the mother can go into spontaneous labour provided that the first twin is lying longitudinally. It is wise to have an intravenous line running. Labour usually proceeds rapidly; although each fetus is small, the total content of the uterus is large. The fetal heart rates of each twin should be monitored separately; some cardiotocographs allow this to be shown on a single chart. An anaesthetist should be present at delivery, and an epidural makes delivery of the second twin easier if there is a malpresentation (which occurs in 5-15% of cases). Paediatricians also should be present at the second stage of labour.

After the first twin is delivered, the cord should be clamped and the lie of the second twin assessed carefully. This can be done clinically, but ultrasound scanning is more reliable. If the lie is not longitudinal, it should be made so by an external cephalic or internal podalic version. Unless uterine contractions return within 15 minutes, stimulation of the uterus with dilute oxytocin should be started, with an aim of delivering the second twin 25-45 minutes after the first. If there is any difficulty in delivery of the second twin, or if this twin develops a bradycardia, a vacuum extraction (in a cephalic presentation) or a breech extraction, if the fetus is lying the other way, can be performed. Internal podalic version and breech extraction is usually easy in this situation. It is not necessary to resort automatically to a caesarean section.

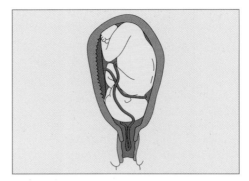

Prolapsed cord into the vagina after membrane rupture with a high head

---

Shoulder dystocia: best delivery method

- Flex and abduct the mother's thighs as much as possible (the McRoberts procedure) and then depress the baby's head towards the mother's anus, with an assistant applying suprapubic pressure
- If this does not work, then manual rotation of the baby through 180° by vaginal and abdominal pressure may succeed
- Cleidotomy or symphysiotomy is the last resort and should be attempted only by an experienced obstetrician

---

Multiple births in United Kingdom, 1995

Type of multiple birth	No of multiple births (rate per 1000 maternities*)	Ratio of multiple to singleton births
Twins	9 889 (13.6)	1:73
Triplets	318 (0.4)	1:2282
Quadruplets	10 (0.0001)	1:72 563
Total	10 217 (14.0)	1:71

Data supplied by Multiple Births Foundation.

*A maternity is any pregnancy that results in the birth of at least one baby; the total number of maternities in 1995 was 725 638.

Conclusions

- Women with a fetus with an abnormal presentation or position should be transferred to hospital for the best care
- Problem cases should be anticipated
- Emergencies during an apparently normal labour need the immediate attention of a skilled obstetrician
- Prepared protocols ensure that all members of the labour suite team know their function and what should be done

---

Key references

- Johnstone F, Myerscough P. Shoulder dystocia. *Br J Obstet Gynaecol* 1998;105:811-5.
- Hofmeyr J. Planned elective caesarean section for term breech. In: Cochrane Collaboration. *Cochrane Library*. Issue 4. Oxford: Update Software, 1997.

9 Operative delivery

Geoffrey Chamberlain, Philip Steer

In Britain all operative deliveries are now performed in a hospital. Caesarean sections must take place in hospital, but the National Birthday Trust's 1994 survey of home births reported that all ventouse and low forceps deliveries also took place in hospital (Chamberlain, 1997). However, not only obstetricians have to know about these deliveries—general practitioners and midwives need to know too, so that they can brief women and prepare to deal with any complications that may arise.

An operative delivery is performed if a spontaneous birth is judged to pose a greater risk to mother or child than an assisted one. Operations are divided into abdominal methods (caesarean section) and vaginal assisted deliveries (forceps delivery and vacuum extraction).

Preparations for operative delivery

- Discuss operative delivery with the woman and her partner (if time is short, at least outline what will happen)
- Follow the woman's wishes—no operative delivery can proceed without her consent even if the doctors think that the baby will die if it is not done
- Get written consent for all procedures if possible
- A paediatrician should attend any delivery where problems are anticipated; local guidelines should be drawn up and followed for all operative deliveries

---

Caesarean section

Use

The frequency of this operation in Britain has increased from about 5% in 1930 to about 16% now. In a survey of 327 obstetricians by Savage et al in Great Britain in the early 1990s, the main reason reported for this rise (cited by 48% of respondents) was fear of litigation (defensive medicine).

In the United States, where the rate for caesarean sections is even higher, close scrutiny by peers and consumer groups has been associated with a reduction; the same may happen in Britain. Even in Britain, the rates vary widely between units.

Indications

The only absolute indications for caesarean section are cephalopelvic disproportion and major degrees of placenta praevia. The rest demand a judgment by the obstetrician that the risk of vaginal delivery exceeds the risk of the operation or sometimes that the mother's perception is that it does.

Caesarean sections are often carried out for debatable indications—for example, breech presentation after 34 weeks. The safety of vaginal birth in these situations often depends on the skill of the birth attendants. Recent evidence shows that perinatal mortality is increased at night and at weekends, when senior staff are less readily available, and is even higher in August and in February, when new resident staff arrive (*Maternity Statistics*, 1997). With shorter training hours and less exposure to difficult vaginal deliveries, deskilling of obstetricians has occurred, so that an elective caesarean section during office hours may well be seen to be safer than a difficult vaginal birth performed out of hours by a junior doctor.

The use of repeat caesarean section depends on the indication for the first caesarean section. If the indication was

---

NHS hospital deliveries England, 1980-94 (from *NHS Maternity Statistics England*, 1997)

Type of delivery	% of all deliveries
Normal	
Vertex	71.5
Breech	0.9
Other	1.3
Total	73.7
Assisted vaginal	
Forceps:	
Low	3.3
Other	2.4
Vacuum	4.8
Total	10.6
Caesarean section	
Elective	6.5
Emergency	9.0
Total	15.5
Other	0.2

Home deliveries made up 2% of all deliveries, and all were normal births

---

Indications for caesarean section

Cephalopelvic disproportion—When it is obvious either antenatally or in the early stages of labour that the fetus, presenting by the head, is not going to pass through the pelvis

Relative cephalopelvic disproportion—The fetus descends initially during labour but is then arrested, possibly due to a malposition such as occipito-posterior

Placenta praevia—Particularly if it is overlapping the internal os

Fetal distress—In the first stage of labour

Prolapsed cord

To avoid fetal hypoxia—When there is poor perfusion of the placental bed (for example, pre-eclampsia)

Malpositions—For example, brow

Malpresentations—For example, transverse lie, breech

Bad obstetric history

Maternal request

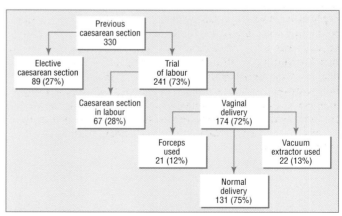

Delivery in one hospital (with low primary caesarean section rate) among 330 women who had previously had caesarean section, 1995

31

recurrent—such as a small pelvis—this demands a repeat caesarean section. If however, the indication was not necessarily recurrent—such as fetal distress—vaginal delivery can be tried. In Britain about two thirds of women who have had a caesarean section try a vaginal delivery in their next pregnancy, and in about two thirds of these a vaginal delivery is successful.

Procedure

How to perform a caesarean section is best learned in the operating theatre with a mentor. It must be learned through practice, with skilled teachers assisting. What follows here is a brief account of the operation—to show what happens, not how to do it. The usual approach is through a transverse lower abdominal incision (Pfannenstiel's incision). Having opened the abdomen carefully, the obstetrician exposes the lower segment of the uterus. The visceral peritoneum is incised and the bladder pushed down, having previously been drained with an indwelling catheter. The uterus is opened slowly with a transverse incision, and when the bulge of membranes appears, this is pricked and the amniotic sac is opened fully with a finger from each side.

The baby is delivered; if presentation is by the head, sometimes a pair of short obstetric forceps is helpful. With a breech presentation, the legs are brought down and a modified breech extraction is performed. If the lie is transverse, the obstetrician aims to bring down the legs to move the baby into a breech position. Care has to be taken not to bring down an arm.

Syntometrine is given, and the placenta is delivered by controlled cord traction. Manual removal increases the blood loss and should be performed only if the placenta is adherent. The uterus is closed in layers, as is the abdominal wall.

A vertical uterine incision used to be used but is now done only in exceptional circumstances: if the lower segment is unapproachable because of fibroids; if there is a transverse fetal lie with the back inferior; or if the lower segment is not formed (for example, before 28 weeks' gestation). Such an incision means that future births will probably be by caesarean as rupture of the vertical scar in the next labour is many times more common than rupture of a transverse scar, and a rupture in the upper segment bleeds much more than one in the lower segment.

Many caesarean sections are now performed under a regional block—spinal (fastest and densest block) or an epidural (allows postoperative top ups for continuing pain relief). General anaesthesia is best avoided as the incidence of complications postoperatively is substantially higher (aspiration of stomach contents, chest infections, and thrombosis). The main indications for general anaesthesia are maternal anxiety, an operation that is likely to be complicated, or, in an emergency, when there is insufficient time to establish an epidural or spinal block.

Complications

Currently, most women receive antibiotic prophylaxis as many studies have shown this to be cost effective, and subcutaneous heparin is increasingly given to prevent venous thrombosis and embolism. The latter is mandatory if there are additional risk factors, such as pre-eclampsia, prolonged inactivity, or obesity.

Postoperative care

The woman usually rises from her bed in the first 24 hours to exercise her legs and to go to the lavatory. The wound is commonly closed with clips or subcuticular prolene; the former can be removed on the fourth day, and this is now the peak time for discharge from hospital. Pain, lack of sleep, and

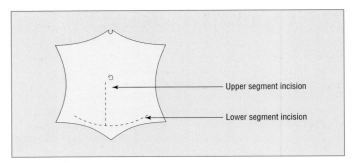

Skin incisions used for caesarean section: for lower segment operation, a gently curved Pfannenstiel's incision following the Langer's lines in the skin, about 3 cm above the pubis in the centre; for classic upper segment operation, a vertical right paramedian incision from level of umbilicus to 3 cm above symphysis pubis

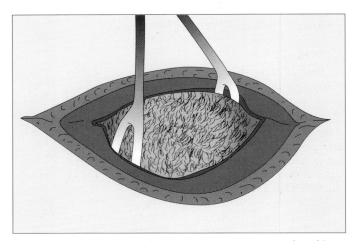

Extracting the fetal head through a lower segment caesarean section with Wrigley's forceps

Complications of caesarean section

Haemorrhage
● Worst from the angles of the uterine incision or with placenta previa

Infection
● Prophylactic antibiotics usually given for caesarean sections, particularly if done after the membranes have ruptured

Thrombosis
● Eight times the risk than after vaginal deliveries
● Commonly occurs in the leg or pelvic veins
● Risk that the thrombus may embolise to a pulmonary vessel
● Prophylactic anticoagulation is given, particularly for those at highest risk (age over 35, anaemia, history of thrombosis, obese)

Ileus
● Mild ileus may last for a day after operation
● Treat conservatively with intravenous fluids and no oral fluids until the mother has passed flatus

difficulty with establishing breast feeding must all be watched for and dealt with appropriately. A discussion on the next day with the parents explaining why the caesarean was necessary is useful as many women have poor recollection of emergency events. Women should be assessed for any resulting psychological morbidity and appropriate help offered.

Forceps

A pair of curved blades can secure a purchase on the rounded head and so apply traction to alter the speed of progress. Usually this is to hasten delivery, but occasionally it is to slow it down, as when delivering the after-coming head in a breech delivery.

Use

Forceps deliveries are performed in 5-10% of deliveries depending on the indication, the availability of trained obstetricians, and the population served. In Britain, use of vacuum extraction is now greater than use of forceps because of reduced maternal trauma; both forms of vaginal delivery, however, are giving way to caesarean section.

Indications

All indications are relative and depend on the facilities for diagnosis and the attitudes of the professional staff.

Types of instruments

There are two types—those with a pelvic curve for extraction, and those without, Kielland's forceps for rotation and extraction; Simpson's forceps are for midcavity assisted delivery without the need for rotation when the maximum diameter of the fetal head is about 5-8 cm above the vulva. Short forceps (Wrigley's) are for low extraction when the maximum diameter is about 2.5 cm above the vulva. These were designed for use by general practitioner obstetricians, with the safety feature that they could not reach high into the pelvis for they are shorter.

Procedure

How to use forceps is again best learned by watching and doing the procedure under skilled tutelage. The woman should receive an explanation of what will happen.

The bladder is catheterised, and regional anaesthesia is given. Each blade is slipped beside the fetal head, the vagina being guarded by the operator's hand. When correctly sited, the handles should lock, and gentle traction in the correct line of pull will help delivery. An episiotomy is usually required to achieve a line of pull sufficiently posterior. Once the head is crowned, the blades can be removed and the rest of the baby delivered normally.

Criteria to be fulfilled before forceps delivery

Cervix must be fully dilated—attempts to apply forceps blades with an undilated cervix will lead to much trauma and bleeding without successful delivery

Bladder must be empty—if necessary emptied with a catheter. This prevents trauma and subsequent lack of bladder sensation

Membranes should be ruptured

No obvious bar exists to delivery, such as disproportion

Episiotomy should usually be performed to allow space for the posterior pull

Analgesia—some form should be used: lignocaine pudendal block with infiltration to the vulva is sometimes enough for a mid-cavity forceps; more anaesthesia (epidural or spinal) is usually needed for rotation forceps

---

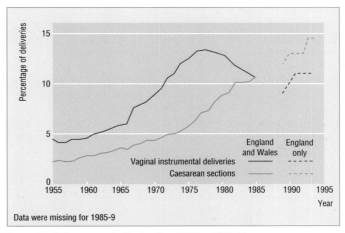

Operative delivery rates in England and Wales, 1955-95

Data were missing for 1985-9

Indications for using obstetric forceps

- Fetal distress in second stage of labour
- Maternal distress in second stage of labour
- Lack of advance in second stage of labour
- Prophylactic shortening of second stage—for example, in heart disease
- Control of after-coming head in a breech delivery

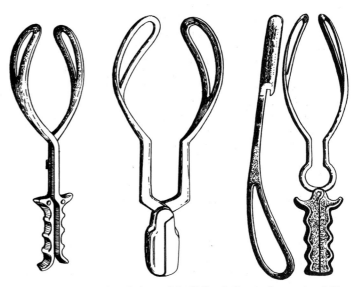

Types of forceps used in Britain: straight Kielland's forceps for rotation (left); curved Wrigley's forceps for lower cavity traction (centre); curved Simpson's forceps for mid-cavity traction (right)

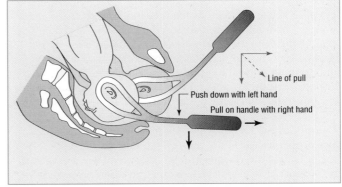

Correct line for pull of forceps. The line of pull is the resultant of two lines of forces in mid-cavity. As the head descends, the line of pull needs to become more anterior to negotiate the pelvic curve

Complications

A perineal tear may extend from the episiotomy, leading to:
- Damage to the vagina or rectum;
- Bleeding;
- Reflex retention of urine.

Fetal scalp haematoma may occur. If the blades are applied improperly, intracranial haemorrhage can follow. Temporary facial palsy may be due to pressure on the facial nerve in front of the fetal ear where the nerve is unprotected. Permanent facial palsy is rare and probably due to a developmental abnormality.

Vacuum extractor

Vacuum extraction is fast becoming the method of choice for vaginal assisted delivery. A negative pressure raises an overhang of soft tissues in the rim of the metal cap, so that the pull is on the overhang of the fetal scalp at this edge. Silastic caps give more surface area applied to the scalp.

Use

Vacuum extraction is widely used in Europe, increasingly in Britain, and least in the United States. Depending on the skills of the obstetrician, about 5% of deliveries can be assisted by a vacuum extractor.

Indications

The vacuum extractor can be used in the first stage of labour before dilatation of the cervix, although this is now rarely done and is potentially dangerous for less experienced staff. Vacuum extractors have a safety factor—they will come off if too much traction is applied, so they are not useful with even mild disproportion. They require less maternal analgesia and cause less maternal trauma than forceps, but the incidence of scalp trauma in the baby is increased; they should not be used before 34 weeks' gestational age because of the softer fetal head.

Types of instruments

The conventional vacuum extractor has a metal cap of 60 mm, 50 mm, or 40 mm diameter. The negative pressure is usually applied by a foot controlled vacuum pump. There are also Silastic caps, which cause fewer abrasions but exert less traction. They have irregularities of their inner surface for a better grip of the scalp, which is particularly useful for helping rotation through the birth canal.

Procedure

Vacuum extraction is best learned by watching and helping a more senior operator. In essence, the largest cap possible should be used. It should lie flat against the fetal head. The pressure is reduced so that it is below 0.8 kg/cm² atmospheric pressure. A check should be made that no part of the vaginal wall (or, if not fully dilated, the cervix) has been sucked in. The cap is held on to the head with the left hand as traction is applied with the right hand. The correct line of pull is very important to prevent the cap coming off and the head not flexing correctly. An early episiotomy is often required to allow the pull to be sufficiently posterior.

Complications

Damage can occur to the cervix if not fully dilated and to the vaginal wall. Such damage can be prevented by checking that no redundant wall is sucked into the cap when the negative pressure has been raised. Haematoma of the baby's scalp sometimes occurs but usually disappears in a week; scalp abrasions may also occur but usually heal readily.

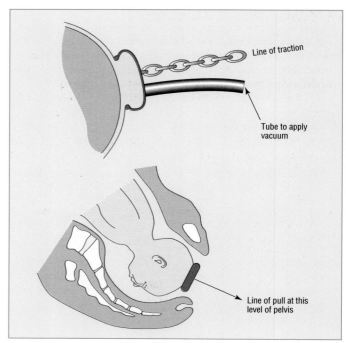

Line of traction

Tube to apply vacuum

Line of pull at this level of pelvis

Vacuum extraction. Top: Chignon of loose skin raised by vacuum; note that pull is on the overhang. Bottom: Line of traction in the mid-cavity is more posterior than would be expected, so early episiotomy is indicated

---

Indications for use of vacuum extractor (ventouse)

First stage of labour (rarely)
- Fetal distress after cervix is 8 cm dilated in a multiparous woman
- Lack of advance after 8 cm dilation in a multiparous woman

Second stage of labour (commonly)
- Lack of advance—often with occipito-posterior or occipito-transverse position
- After an epidural has relaxed the pelvic floor
- If the mother is tired
- If the head of a second twin is high

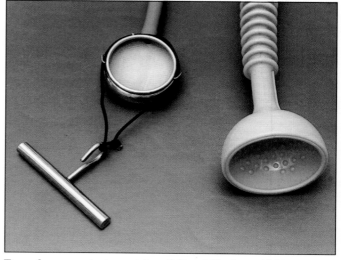

Types of vacuum extractor: metal cap (left) and Silastic cap (right)

Genital tract trauma

The perineal skin does not stretch as well as the vagina, probably owing to the increased fibrous content of the skin compared with vaginal epithelium. Perineal tears are classically divided into three grades according to severity.

If the perineum seems to be splitting, an episiotomy is often performed to limit the damage. Episiotomies are not done routinely now but for specific indications; in Britain the rate varies from 15% to 40% of women, depending on the hospital.

An episiotomy should always be done under anaesthesia (at least 1% lignocaine infiltration). In Britain an episiotomy is usually mediolateral so that if the incision extends, it does not run into the anus. Episiotomies are usually repaired by trained midwives, preferably the one who performed the episiotomy.

Occasionally the episiotomy will extend at its upper end in the vaginal tissues into one of the fornices. This must be checked for carefully when repairing. It is important for haemostasis to put in at least one stitch above the highest point of the cut or tear to occlude vessels coming in from above.

> **Operative deliveries are performed by trained obstetricians, but the events leading up to and following such deliveries are in the care of many other health workers, all of whom should be knowledgeable about the subject**

Key references

- Steer PJ. Caesarean section—an evolving procedure. *Br J Obstet Gynaecol* 1998;105:1052-5.
- Chamberlain G, Wraight A, Crowley P. *Home Births*. London: Parthenon, 1997:67.
- Drife J. Choice and instrumental delivery. *Br J Obstet Gynaecol* 1996;103:608-11.
- Enkin M, Keirse M, Renfrew M, Neilson J. *Effective care in pregnancy and childbirth*. Oxford: Oxford University Press, 1995:284-93.
- Grant A, Penn ZJ, Steer PJ. Elective or selective caesarean delivery of the small baby? A systematic review of the controlled trials. *Br J Obstet Gynaecol* 1996;103:1197-200.
- Kuit J, Eppinga H, Wakenburg H, Huikeshaven J. A randomised comparison of vacuum extraction delivery with a rigid or pliable cap. *Obstet Gynecol* 1993;82:280-4.
- Department of Health. *NHS maternity statistics 1980-1994*. London: Stationery Office, 1997.
- O'Driscol K, Meagher D, Boylan P. *Active management of labour*. New York: Mosby, 1995.
- Savage W, Trancome C. Why caesarean section? *Br J Obstet Gynaecol* 1993;100:493-6.

Staging of degrees of perineal tear in order of severity

Stage 1: Skin of fourchette or vagina only
Stage 2: Skin and superficial perineal muscles
Stage 3: Anal muscles and sphincter involved*

*In the United States, stage 3 is confined to tears to the anal margin, while involvement of the sphincter and rectal mucosa becomes stage 4

Indications for episiotomy

- To speed the later part of the second stage of labour in the presence of fetal distress
- To open up posterior areas to allow the correct line of traction at forceps or vacuum extraction
- To overcome a perineum that is rigid and delaying the last part of delivery
- If there is likely to be a major perineal tear, an episiotomy may prevent it and may be easier to repair

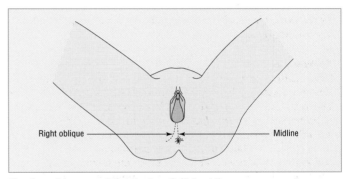

Sites for episiotomy: midline heals well; right oblique curves away from anus

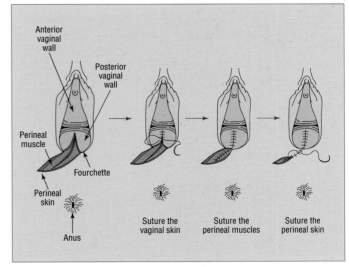

Repair of episiotomy. A recent trial has shown that suturing of the skin is not necessary provided that the muscle layer is well closed

The data in the figure showing delivery in women who had previously had a caesarean section were provided by the master of the National Maternity Hospital, Dublin. The graph on operative delivery rates in England and Wales is adapted from one prepared by Alison Macfarlane based on data from the maternity hospital inpatient inquiry and hospital episodes statistics.

10 Obstetric emergencies

Geoffrey Chamberlain, Philip Steer

The management of emergencies is usually the responsibility of hospital obstetricians. As more maternity care is now given in the community, however, midwives, general practitioners, and paramedics may be involved and must know the outlines of management of emergencies and the possible side effects. If such a situation occurs outside the hospital then arrangements must be made to transport the woman to the obstetric unit, safely and promptly.

All emergency protocols should have been considered beforehand and mutually agreed by obstetricians, midwives, general practitioners, and paramedics. Everybody then knows their immediate priority, and hazards to the woman can be minimised.

Abruption of the placenta

An abruption is a death threat to the fetus and a hazard to the mother. When the placenta separates from its bed (probably because of the rupture of a malformed blood vessel), the damage to the fetus follows not just because of the barrier that the clot makes between the placental bed and villi but also because the release of prostaglandins causes a major degree of uterine spasm. This interferes with perfusion of the placenta which remains attached. Blood tracking into the myometrium often goes as far as the peritoneum over the uterus, causing much pain and shock, with spasm of the uterine muscle.

In major degrees of placental abruption the woman is shocked well beyond the apparent amount of blood loss and needs urgent transport into hospital. A wide bore intravenous line should be set up and blood sent for cross matching of at least six units of blood. Until this blood arrives, other plasma expanding fluids, such as Haemaccel, should be used.

If the fetus is still alive and gestation sufficiently advanced, caesarean section is the best management. However, if the fetus is dead, conservative management can be pursued provided that the woman does not continue deteriorating—for example, by developing a coagulopathy. Most women with a severe abruption that kills the fetus will go into spontaneous labour soon and have an easy delivery, but caesarean section is occasionally necessary for maternal indications alone. Treatment must be aimed at the shock and at preventing disseminated intravascular coagulopathy.

Half the time the placenta is implanted on the anterior wall of the uterus, but if it is posterior, when the abruption is less painful and not so severe that the mother is shocked; the fetus will still be at risk, however. Diagnosis in these cases is by recognition of the excessively frequent contractions produced by the prostaglandin release and the abnormal pattern of the fetal heart rate secondary to fetal hypoxia; these are best shown with cardiotocography, a priority investigation in all women admitted with abdominal pain in pregnancy.

Placenta praevia

The blastocyst occasionally implants in the lower part of the uterus. Stretching and thinning of the uterine muscle of the lower segment in the third trimester may sheer off part of the placental attachment. This is accompanied by painless bleeding.

> The first principles of dealing with obstetric emergencies are the same as for any emergency (see to the airway, breathing, and circulation), but remember that in obstetrics there are two patients; the fetus is very vulnerable to maternal hypoxia

---

Clinical features of abruption of the placenta

Symptoms
- Abdominal pain
- Severe shock with symptoms beyond the vaginal blood loss
- Vaginal bleeding—usually old blood

Signs
- Shock
- Spasm of uterus—described as woody
- Tender uterus
- Fetal parts hard to feel
- Often no fetal heart beats are present

Emergency treatment of abruption

Treat the shock
- Give oxygen
- Insert large bore intravenous lines
- Arrange a cross match of 6 units of blood
- Give morphine (if fetus dead)

Deliver the fetus
- By caesarean section (if fetus is alive and gestation is mature)
- By rupturing membranes (if cervix is ripe or fetus is dead)

Treat disseminated intravascular coagulopathy
- Urgent haematological consultation
- Check platelet count
- Give cryoprecipitate (fresh frozen plasma)
- Transfuse with fresh blood if available

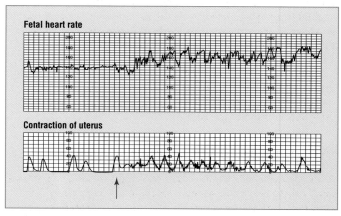

Cardiotocograph during an abruption of placenta (arrow indicates sudden abdominal pain)

Often the fetus is not affected by the first small bleeds, but they should be taken seriously for there is a risk that the mother could have a much larger bleed. Women with bright red, painless vaginal bleeding in later pregnancy are considered to have placenta praevia until proved otherwise and should be admitted to hospital. Vaginal ultrasound examination is the best technique for investigating possible placenta praevia, but, although it has a high sensitivity and specificity for central placenta praevia in the third trimester, it is much less precise in the late second trimester or for marginal placenta praevia. Management should therefore always be based on appropriate clinical judgment.

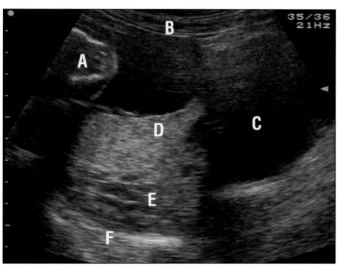

Ultrasound picture of placenta praevia. A=fetal head; B=anterior uterine wall; C=full bladder; D=placenta; E=placental lakes; F=cervical canal

If placenta praevia is confirmed the woman should stay in hospital for at least 48 hours after the bleeding has stopped. Management is conservative, even to the level of giving blood transfusions for severe bleeds, until the fetus is mature (at about 36 weeks). Studies do not show any benefit in keeping women in hospital until delivery, provided that they have a telephone at home and live close enough to the hospital to be brought in by the emergency services within 20 minutes if they start bleeding again (Love et al, 1996). Unless it is very obvious—for example, a complete placenta praevia on ultrasound examination, together with a transverse lie of the fetus—placenta praevia is sometimes confirmed by examination under general anaesthesia in theatre, proceeding in most instances to caesarean section performed by a senior obstetrician. Occasionally, if the placenta is anterior and just enplanting in the lower segment, the membranes may be ruptured and a vaginal delivery expected, as the head coming down into the mother's pelvis will compress the bleeding placental bed against the back of the pubis symphysis. The same cannot be said for any degree of posterior placenta praevia.

After delivery, a postpartum haemorrhage is likely because the placental bed is situated over less well contracting uterine muscle and may well bleed despite oxytocic stimulation. This often requires blood transfusion.

Postpartum haemorrhage

After a normal delivery a woman commonly loses up to 300 ml of blood. As her blood volume has increased because of fluid retention during pregnancy, this is a loss which can be coped with readily. However, a loss of >500 ml measured clinically in the first 24 hours is considered to be a primary postpartum

Clinical aspects of placenta praevia
Symptoms
- Vaginal bleeding—bright red, painless, recurrent
Signs
- Soft, non-tender uterus
- Easy to feel fetus—often high head, breech, or transverse lie
- No fetal distress

Do not do a digital vaginal examination
A speculum examination once a woman is an inpatient to exclude any local bleeding is acceptable

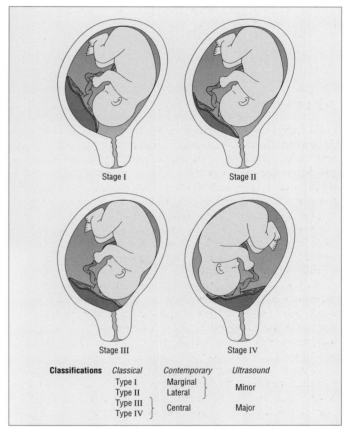

Four stages of severity of placenta praevia: I—placenta encroaches on lower segment but does not reach internal os; II—placenta reaches internal os but does not cover it; III—placenta covers internal os before dilatation but not when dilated; IV—placenta completely covers internal os even when dilated

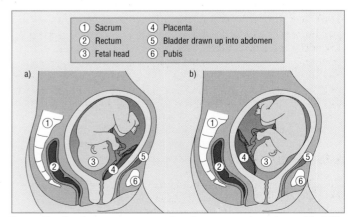

Descending head can compress anterior placenta praevia against pubis (left) but not posterior sited placenta (right) as too much soft tissue intervenes

haemorrhage. Blood loss is commonly underestimated by the attending practitioners. The mother should be watched carefully and treatments given to prevent any further loss.

If the uterus has not contracted firmly, manual stimulation may work by rubbing up a contraction, and a further oxytocic is given. If the placenta is incomplete the uterine cavity is explored for the remaining lobules whose presence in the uterine cavity may prevent the organ contracting down. If neither of these conditions exists, trauma to the lower uterus, cervix, or upper vagina may be the cause of the bleeding. Such traumas should be looked for (under GA with a good light) and sutured appropriately. A rare cause of continuing primary postpartum haemorrhage is a rupture of the uterus. This needs diagnosis and treatment with either hysterectomy or abdominal resuturing.

After the first 24 hours, any bleeding is a secondary postpartum haemorrhage. It is commonly associated with infection, which should be treated vigorously with intravenous antibiotics. If it persists, suction evacuation of the uterus should be undertaken by a senior obstetrician; perforation of the soft uterus is a major risk in this situation.

A complication of severe and prolonged blood loss is a consumptive coagulopathy, when the mother's blood does not clot owing to interference with the clotting cascade. The continuing cooperation of a senior haematologist is essential. The mother continues to bleed not just from the placental bed but from other sites in the body. This needs firm and prompt correction so that full coagulation can be restored. Giving cryoprecipitate (frozen precipitate) provides many of the missing components.

Amniotic fluid embolism

Occasionally, when the uterus is contracting strongly and there is an opening between the amniotic sac and the uterine veins, a bolus of amniotic fluid is pumped into the circulation. This passes through the heart, and an accumulation of amniotic cells becomes trapped in the pulmonary circulation. The amniotic fluid may cause local disseminated intravascular coagulation, which may spread. This rare condition can occur late in the last trimester or during labour.

Amniotic fluid embolism used to be diagnosed on histology only after a postmortem examination but is now sometimes diagnosed before death. The symptoms include collapse while having strong contractions, shock without any blood loss, sudden dyspnoea, and the production of frothy sputum. Treatment is supportive, with steroids, intravenous plasma expansion, and urgent delivery. This obstetric emergency is rare and has a bad prognosis for both mother and fetus, usually due to delay in diagnosis.

Inversion of uterus

Very rarely, if misapplied pressure has been used on the uterine fundus or traction on the cord of a non-separated placenta in a multiparous woman, the uterus can dimple and invert. This is a very shocking event as the fundus turns inside out and goes through the cervix into the vagina. Treatment requires an experienced obstetrician, who will try to return the uterus under general anaesthesia. This can be very difficult.

Infection

After delivery the genital tract has several sites of potential ingress of bacteria. The placental bed itself is a large raw area,

Management of primary postpartum haemorrhage

Preventive
- Intramuscular oxytocin at the end of the second stage of labour

Curative
- Repeat oxytocic administration
- Rub up a contraction
- Check completeness of the placenta—if it is not delivered or a lobule is missing, prepare for manual removal
- Bimanual compression
- Intramyometrial prostaglandin E_2 or carboprost
- Surgical ligation—uterine arteries, internal iliac arteries, or braces (Lynch) suture of uterus
- Hysterectomy

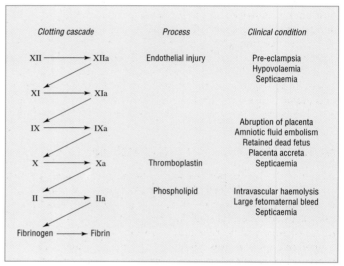

Mechanisms of blood clotting, and some of the clinical conditions that act at various points of the cascade to interfere with clotting

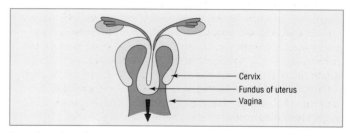

Acute inversion of uterus

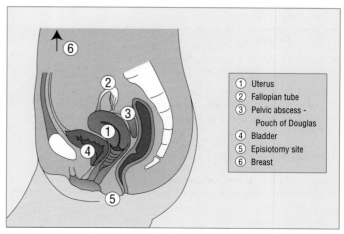

Commonest sites of postpartum infection

and ascending infection from the lower genital tract may be assisted by previous intrauterine procedures—for example, forceps delivery. Infection of the cervix or, uncommonly, of the episiotomy site, may also occur; the breast can also be a site of infection in the puerperium.

Psychological conditions

Pregnancy and childbirth are times of high psychological stimulation. Any pre-existing psychological disorder may be exaggerated at this time and requires treatment. Many women go through mood swings (blues) in relation to childbirth, which can usually be managed by sympathetic support. If postnatal depression persists for a week or so, mild antidepressants may be needed, and the Edinburgh postnatal depression questionnaire may be helpful in diagnosing the condition. If the condition continues, formal psychiatric help is needed.

At the extreme of the spectrum of disease a puerperal psychosis may occur; both the mother and her baby should be admitted to a dedicated maternity/psychiatric unit as both are at risk. Here the mother can have expert psychiatric nursing and medical care while looking after her own baby. There is a 25% risk of recurrence in a future pregnancy.

Stillbirth and intrauterine death

In Britain 3-4 babies per 1000 are stillborn and another 3-4 per 1000 die in the first week of life. The grief reactions in both the woman and her partner need careful management by the midwifery and medical staff. The couple may go through a phase of anger; all hospital and community staff should be trained to cope with this. Midwifery and medical staff must be prepared to listen and offer their sympathies without attributing blame.

Parents should be encouraged to agree to a postmortem examination of the fetus and placenta by a skilled paediatric pathologist. Getting permission for this from the couple requires sensitivity. If a full postmortem examination is declined, a limited examination of the baby may be acceptable (x ray examination, computed tomography, blood samples from the heart area for chromosome analysis, and bacteriological swabbing of the relevant areas of the body).

Cultural attitudes of the parents influence these decisions and must be respected. It is probable that the couple will not object to full histological examination of the placenta.

Treating infections

- Infections manifest themselves by local inflammation (swelling and tenderness) and a raised temperature
- Treatment is local heat to the area, analgesia, and broad spectrum antibiotics until the results of bacteriological swabs are available
- Co-amoxiclav and erythromycin are both good choices because they deal with penicillinase-producing staphylococci and streptococci, especially those of group B
- Metronidazole is often added for uterine infections
- If the infection persists, anaemia may follow, which may ultimately require a blood transfusion

Three levels of psychiatric state associated with childbirth

Postpartum blues (1 in 5 mothers)
- Transient and treatable by reassurance

Puerpural depression (1 in 10 mothers)
- Low mood, lack of energy, guilt, irritability, and insomnia
- Treated by counselling (midwives and health visitors)
- Antidepressants—refer to GP if depression continues

Puerpural psychosis (1 in 500 mothers)
- Affective, depressive, or manic behaviour; insomnia; confusion; perplexity
- Refer to psychiatrist and admit to mother and baby unit

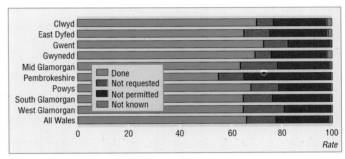

Example of health district data on frequency of perinatal postmortem examinations and consent sought (data from the Welsh confidential inquiry into stillbirths and deaths in infancy, 1996)

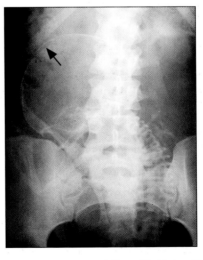

Radiograph of intrauterine death showing overlap of cranial bones after collapse of fetal skull. Ultrasound changes after death are of a more functional nature (lack of movements or fetal heart beat) but not so helpful at showing structural changes

Professor Robert Kendell provided help with the section on psychological and psychiatric conditions. The table showing presenting symptoms in fulminating pre-eclampsia is adapted from Sibai et al (*Am J Obstet Gynecol* 1993;169:1000-6). The cardiotocograph is adapted from Ingemarsson et al (*Fetal heart rate monitoring*. Oxford: Oxford Medical Publications, 1993). The drawing showing mechanisms of blood clotting is adapted from Letsky (*Obstetrics*. London: Churchill Livingstone, 1995).

Key references

- Love C, Wallace E. Pregnancies complicated by placenta praevia: what is appropriate management? *Br J Obstet Gynaecol* 1996;103:864-7.
- Department of Health. *Confidential enquiries into maternal death (1988-1990)*. London: HMSO, 1994:43-6.
- Douglas K, Redman C. Eclampsia in the United Kingdom. *BMJ* 1994;309:1395-400.
- James D, Steer P, Weiner C, Gonik B. *High risk obstetrics*. London: Saunders, 1999.
- SANDS (Stillbirth and Neonatal Death Society). *Guidelines for professionals*. London: SANDS, 1991.

11 Care of the newborn in the delivery room

Patricia Hamilton

It is the duty of those attending a delivery to ensure that the baby is given any resuscitation that may be needed and to do a brief external examination of the baby to exclude immediate problems. Any risk factors for sepsis or other neonatal problems should be communicated to the paediatricians.

Resuscitation

Most newborn babies will establish normal breathing spontaneously. They need only attention to the maintenance of their temperature and perhaps gentle stimulation to start breathing; some may need suction of the airway, and a few will need assisted lung inflation via a mask. Fewer still need tracheal intubation, and very few indeed will need external chest compression and intervention with drugs.

Successful resuscitation requires the coordinated efforts of a professional team. All midwives, neonatal nurses, and doctors who might attend a delivery should be competent in lung inflation and ventilation via a mask. Tracheal intubation should be undertaken only by those who have been trained in its use and who have sufficient practice to maintain the skill.

Physiology

The first few breaths overcome the surface tension within the lung, drive any residual fluid from the alveoli into the circulation, and fill the lungs with air. Once the initial opening pressure has been achieved, subsequent breaths need not be so forceful.

In utero little blood flows to the lungs because of high resistance in the pulmonary circulation and lower resistance to flow into the aorta and placenta. Resistance to flow into the pulmonary circulation rapidly falls after lung expansion, and as a result the blood leaving the right ventricle passes into the pulmonary circulation.

Anticipation of need for resuscitation

Local circumstances will dictate when an appropriately trained person should be called to stand by at a delivery. Someone experienced in resuscitation (with an assistant) should be present to deal with certain situations.

Before delivery it is important to check that the correct equipment is present and functioning properly. The room should be warm, the radiant heat source switched on, and prewarmed towels available. The mother's case notes should be checked for any relevant information, in particular any antenatal diagnosis made, any relevant maternal condition, or any risk factors for infection. Surgical gloves should be worn over clean hands to protect the baby and the attending professional (Royal College of Obstetricians and Gynaecologists, 1990).

The baby should be assessed after birth. Even a vigorous newborn baby may have a marked fall in body temperature if exposed, and should be covered with a warm, dry towel at all times. Most babies will breathe or cry within 90 seconds of birth; suction of the pharynx is not usually necessary, nor is additional oxygen. These babies should be handed direct to the mother.

If the baby is not breathing adequately, the ABC of resuscitation should be followed.

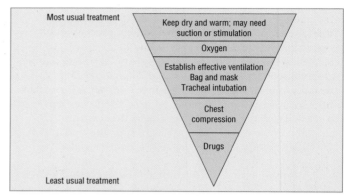

Triangle of resuscitation—relative frequencies and priorities for neonatal resuscitation

At every delivery, wherever it takes place, there should be at least one person who is responsible for giving basic care to the baby, initiating resuscitation if necessary, and summoning more help if needed (British Paediatric Association, 1993)

Conditions in which neonatal resuscitation may be needed*

- Fetal distress
- Thick meconium staining of amniotic fluid
- Vaginal breech deliveries
- Gestation of <32 completed weeks
- Serious congenital abnormality
- Concern of attending staff

*Someone experienced in resuscitation, and an assistant, should be present

Apgar scores in newborn

Sign	Score		
	0	1	2
Heart rate	Nil	<100	>100
Respiratory effort	Absent	Gasping or irregular	Regular or crying
Muscle tone	Flaccid	Some tone	Active
Response to stimulation	None	Grimace	Cry or cough
Colour	White	Blue	Pink centrally

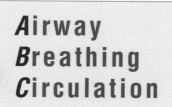

ABC of resuscitation

Airway

The baby should be positioned face upwards with the head supported in the neutral position. If respiratory efforts are vigorous but no breath sounds are heard, the airway may be obstructed. Reposition the baby and gently suck out the mouth and nostrils.

Breathing

If respiratory efforts are shallow or slow and no meconium is present, stimulate gently and offer supplementary oxygen if the baby is cyanosed. If the heart rate is < 100 beats/minute or decreasing, start lung inflation via a mask. If there is no response, prepare to perform tracheal intubation and call for help if necessary.

Circulation

Assess the circulation by evaluating the heart rate and the colour of the baby. Monitor the heart rate by auscultation or palpation of the base of the cord. If it is > 100 beats/minute continue assessment, but if it is < 100 beats/minute and decreasing, start or continue positive pressure ventilation.

If the heart rate is less than 60 beats/minute, start external chest compression and consider drugs and volume expansion.

Positive pressure ventilation

By a face mask

Apply the right size face mask holding the chin gently forward. If using a Y piece ensure that there is a suitable pressure relief valve; if using a resuscitation bag and valve, squeeze the bag slowly with the finger tips.

Ventilate the lungs at a rate of 30-40 breaths per minute. See that the chest wall moves with each inflation and listen for breath and heart sounds.

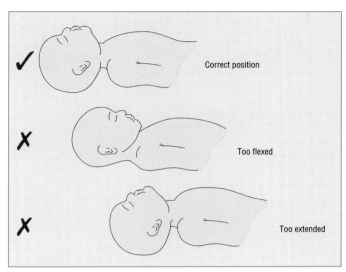

Position of baby for resuscitation

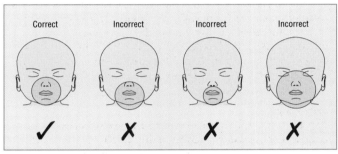

Positive pressure ventilation: correct position and size of face mask

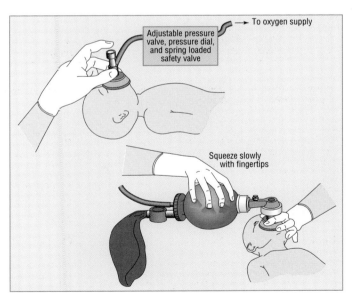

Resuscitation with face mask and Y piece (left) and with bag and mask (right)

Tracheal intubation

Lift the straight bladed laryngoscope upwards and forwards in the direction of the handle and keep the vocal cords in view while inserting an uncuffed tracheal tube. Keep the curve of the tube in the horizontal plane so that the larynx is not obscured. The shoulder of the tube or the intubation mark should be positioned just above the cords.

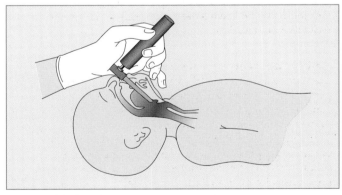

Correct positioning of laryngoscope

Causes of failure to respond to intubation

- Disconnection of equipment
- Tube in oesophagus
- Tube in right main bronchus
- Insufficient inflation pressure
- Pneumothorax
- Pleural effusion
- Diaphragmatic hernia

External chest compression

Place the thumbs over the lower third of the sternum with the hands around the chest, or apply pressure with two fingers. The sternum should be compressed by about 2-3 cm in a term baby at a rate of about 2 compressions per second, and the lungs should be reinflated with oxygen after every 3 compressions.

Drugs and fluids

Adrenaline should be given initially, followed by sodium bicarbonate if necessary. Hypovolaemia should be considered when there is evidence of acute bleeding or poor response to adequate resuscitation. Naloxone should be reserved for the apnoeic baby whose mother has received opiate analgesia 2-4 hours before delivery. It is not a substitute for resuscitation.

Drugs for use in neonatal resuscitation

Adrenaline
Preparation 1 in 10 000 dilution (100 µg/ml)
Dose 1st and 2nd dose 10 µg/kg (0.1 ml/kg); 3rd dose 100 µg/kg
  (1 ml/kg)
Route 1st dose, tracheal tube (provided that lungs are inflated);
  2nd and 3rd doses, umbilical venous catheter

Sodium bicarbonate
Preparation 4.2% (0.5 mmol/ml) or 8.4% (1 mmol/ml) solution with
  equal volume of dextrose
Dose 1-2 mmol/kg (2-4 ml/kg of 4.2% solution) via umbilical venous
  catheter; 2 doses may be given

Volume expanders
Preparations Plasma, or group O Rh negative blood that is not cross
  matched; 4-5% human albumin
Dose 10-20 ml/kg via umbilical venous catheter over 5-10 minutes
  (may be repeated)

Naloxone hydrochloride*
Dose 100 µg/kg (0.25 ml/kg) intramuscularly

*Never give to the baby of an opiate dependent mother

Umbilical venous catheterisation

Injection into a peripheral vein may not be effective, and a catheter should be inserted into the umbilical vein. Blood or other fluid may be given by this route.

Meconium

If the amniotic fluid is lightly stained with meconium and the baby is well it is not necessary to intubate. If there is particulate meconium, aspirate the mouth and nostrils gently as soon as the head is delivered. If the baby is vigorous and pink, intubation is of no benefit and may cause later complications (Linder et al, 1988). If the baby is not vigorous, intubate and aspirate meconium from the trachea by applying suction directly to the tracheal tube while withdrawing and removing the tube or through a wide-bore suction catheter passed down a large tracheal tube. Ventilate the baby when as much meconium as possible has been removed.

Severe congenital abnormality

Fetal abnormalities are usually diagnosed antenatally, and a clear plan of management can be determined in advance. Occasionally, however, a baby will be born with an unexpected severe abnormality. Unless the abnormality is extreme the baby should still be resuscitated until informed decisions about further management can be made.

Very preterm babies

Decisions about resuscitation should be made by an experienced paediatrician to whom this responsibility has been designated. A preterm baby who is failing to establish regular

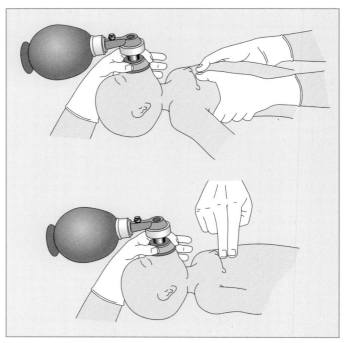

Two methods of external chest compression

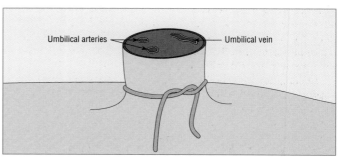

Umbilical cord prepared for venous cannulation

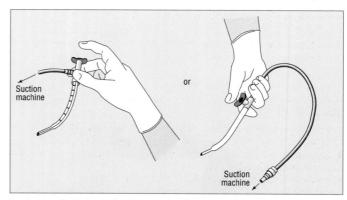

Suction methods for aspiration of meconium

Responsibilities for problems

- Mutually agreed protocols should be prepared in each unit to cover difficult situations:
  Resuscitation of those with severe congenital abnormalities
  Resuscitation of the very preterm baby (< 25 weeks)
- A senior neonatal paediatrician should take part in discussions of each individual case

---

respiration needs more swift support. Very preterm babies who are extremely bruised at delivery or who have been given adrenaline during resuscitation generally have an extremely poor outcome (Sims et al, 1994). If there is doubt, the baby should be resuscitated and taken to the neonatal unit, where decisions about further management can be made.

No response to resuscitation

Resuscitation efforts should usually be abandoned if there is no spontaneous cardiac output after 15 minutes of resuscitation. If the baby has a spontaneous heart rate but is making no respiratory effort, assisted ventilation should continue until further information is available.

Vitamin K

All babies should receive vitamin K at birth to prevent haemorrhagic disease of the newborn. There is currently some controversy over the correct mode of administration, oral or intramuscular (*Drugs and Therapeutics Bulletin*, 1998), and recent guidance has been issued by the Department of Health. Local policies should inform and advise mothers on the arguments for and against the available options.

Examination in delivery room

The examination of babies in the delivery room is currently under review, but at this stage it is appropriate for the deliverer to perform a brief external examination of the baby to exclude major abnormalities. The mother should be aware that her baby will receive a more detailed examination later.

Local guidelines should be available to determine the appropriate gestational age, birth weight, or condition of babies that can be managed on the postnatal wards. The presence of congenital anomaly, maternal diabetes, or risk factors for infection should be taken seriously, and a paediatrician should be informed. It should not be necessary to test the blood glucose concentration in the delivery room.

Every attempt should be made to encourage the mother to breast feed. The baby should, if the mother wishes, be put to the breast immediately after birth or after recovery from any resuscitation.

Finally, it is important to ensure that the parents are fully informed about what has occurred in the delivery room and to complete full records.

Conclusions

- Professionals present at any delivery need the appropriate knowledge and skills to resuscitate a depressed newborn baby
- If positive pressure respiratory assistance is needed, use of a bag and mask will usually suffice
- Intubation requires special skills and regular practice

The text and illustrations on resuscitation are based on *Resuscitation of Babies at Birth* (Royal College of Paediatrics and Child Health and Royal College of Obstetricians and Gynaecologists. London: BMJ Publishing, 1997). A similar account appears in *Current Paediatrics* (1998;8:225-30).

The decision to abandon resuscitation efforts should be taken by an experienced member of staff

---

Examination of the newborn

Area	Examination
Head	Fontanelle, sutures, ears, eyes, face, lip, and palate
Arms	Numbers of fingers, palmer creases
Chest	Listen to heart and lungs
Abdomen	Umbilicus, groins, anus, genitalia
Back	Skin, spine
Legs	Toes, ankles, hips

Conditions to exclude in initial external examination of the newborn

- Birth injuries
- Abnormalities of limbs or digits
- Cyanosis, tachypnoea, or grunting
- Imperforate anus
- Cleft lip or palate
- Significant naevi
- Ambiguous genitalia
- Oesophageal atresia (if polyhydramnios)
- Other obvious congenital abnormality

Key references

- British Paediatric Association. *Neonatal resuscitation.* London: BPA, 1993.
- Royal College of Obstetricians and Gynaecologists. *Working party report on maternity care in obstetrics and gynaecology.* London: Royal College of Obstetricians and Gynaecologists, 1990.
- Linder N, Aranda JV, Tsur M, Matoth I, Yatsiv I, Mandelberg H, et al. Need for endotracheal intubation in meconium stained neonates. *J Pediatr* 1988;112:613-5.
- Sims DG, Heal CA, Bartle SM. Use of adrenaline and atropine in neonatal resuscitation. *Arch Dis Child* 1994;70:F3-10.
- Which vitamin K preparation for the newborn? *Drug Ther Bull* 1998;36:17-9.
- Department of Health. *Vitamin K for newborn babies.* London: DoH, 1998. (PL/CMO/98/3.)

L'ENVOI

This book has been aimed at practitioners of obstetrics and midwifery. It describes briefly the state of the art in the turn of the century with some explanations of the physiology behind patterns of childbirth. In the last hundred years there have been many changes from the dangerous times before the First World War; the hazards of childbirth were reduced with better health of the mothers and the reduction and treatment of sepsis. Blood transfusion came in with World War II and organised antenatal care became widespread, all of which brought benefits. In parallel with this, the greater organisation in training and checking of standards of midwives and doctors followed the formation of their Colleges. Since the 1960s the scientific advances in monitoring and the wider use of safe analgesia were massive advances. In the last twenty years the restoration of the midwife to her correct place in normal delivery and her surveillance against problems has come into its own, and finally the recognition of the mother's place in the self-determination of childbirth has become practised widely.

We hope that this book helps professionals with their training and dealing with problems. Details of treatments are not expanded but the principles are; that is important to make us all think of what we should be doing. We hope it brings safe care to the mother and child and peace of mind to the professional when in doubt.

Index

absolute disproportion 25
active management 8, 25
adrenaline 42, 43
airways, resuscitation 41
alveoli 40
Amnihook 17
amniocentesis 22
amniotic fluid 8, 10, 17, 19, 21, 42
amniotic fluid embolism 19, 38
amniotic membranes 5, 17, 25, 30
amniotomy forceps 17
anaesthesia 14, 32
antenatal steroids 22
antibiotic, prophylaxis 32
aorta 40
Apgar scores 40
aspiration 32
atosiban 22
auscultation 8, 41

bacterial vaginosis 20
baths, warm water 15
birth attendants 7, 8
Bishop's score 5, 17
blastocyst 36
Braxton Hicks contractions 21
breathing, resuscitation 41
breech extraction 30
breech presentations 29
bupivacaine 13

caesarean sections 8, 14, 16, 19, 25, 26,
    29, 30, 33, 36, 37
  complications of 32
  elective 23, 27
  frequency of 31
  indications for 31–2
  postoperative care 32–3
  procedure 32
cardiac disease 26
cardiotocograms 9, 10
cardiotocographs 30, 36
care settings 1–2
catheters, Drew Smythe 17
cephalopelvic disproportion 25, 31
cervical dilatation 5, 8, 21, 24, 25
cervical monitoring 5–6
cervical ripeness 5, 17
cervical ripening 20, 24
Changing Childbirth 1, 3, 8
chest infections 32
chloroform 12
chorioamnionitis 20
chromosome analysis 39
circulation, resuscitation 41
cleidotomy 30
clindamycin 20
clinical errors 11
clotting cascade 38
co-amoxiclav 39
coagulopathy 36, 38
computed tomography 25, 39
comsumptive coagulopathy 38
congenital abnormality, severe 42
congenital heart disease 26

consultant led units 2
contractions, Braxton Hicks 21
corticosteroids 21
Crowley 16
cryoprecipitate 38

delivery, preterm 22–3
delivery positions 7
diamorphine 13
diazepam 26
Doppler fetal heart detector 8
Drew Smythe catheters 17
drugs, use of 6, 42
dyspnoea 38

eclampsia 26
elective caesarean sections 23, 27
electrocardiographic monitoring 26
electronic monitoring 8–10
embolism 32
emergencies
  dealing with 2
  infection 38–9
  obstetric 36–9
Entonox 12, 15
epidural 15, 24, 32
epidural analgesia 9, 13–14, 26, 28
epidural hypotension 26
episiotomy 14, 33, 34, 35
erythromycin 39
examinations, newborn 43
external chest compression 40, 42

face and brow positions 29
face masks, positive pressure ventilation
    41
facial palsy 34
fentanyl 13
fetal acidosis 9, 10
fetal blood sampling 9, 11, 27
fetal circulation 6
fetal head
  descent of 24
  engagement of 25
  rotation of 4, 6
fetal heart rate, monitoring 8–10, 11, 36
fetal hypoxia 9, 10, 11, 25, 36
fetal pulse oximetry 10
fetal scalp haematoma 34
fetal tachycardia 9, 10
forceps
  complications 34
  procedure for 33
  types of 33
  use of 33
  see also amniotomy forceps; Kielland's
    forceps; Kocher's forceps; Wrigley's
    forceps
fundus 38

Gardnerella vaginalis 20
general anaesthesia 14, 32
general practitioner maternity units 1–2
general practitioners 2–3
genital tract trauma 35

glyceryl trinitrate 22

Haemaccel 36
HELLP syndrome 26
heparin 32
HIV 27
home, place of birth 1
HOOP study 7
hospitals, place of birth 1, 2
hydralazine 26
hypovolaemia 42

iatrogenic factors 26
indomethacin 22
induction
  contraindications 17
  incidence 16
  indications 16
  methods of 17–18
  readiness for 16–17
  risks of 19
  success of 18–19
infections 38–9
infrared spectroscopy 10, 11
inhibitors, protease 27
interleukin 1 20
interleukin–6 20
intra-arterial blood pressure
    measurement 26
intracranial haemorrhage 34
intrapartum infection 9
intrauterine death 39
ischial spines 24
isoxuprine hydrochloride 22

Kielland's forceps 14, 28, 33
Kocher's forceps 17, 18

labetalol 26
labour 4
  assessment of mother and fetus 8–11
  preterm 20–3
  slow progress of 24–5, 26
  stages of 5–6
  support for mother 6–7
  use of drugs 6
labour care, general practitioners 2–3
lactate 10, 11
laryngoscope 41
lead professionals 3
legal responsibilities, general
    practitioners 3
lignocaine 14
lung inflation 40

McRoberts procedure 30
magnesium sulphate 26
magnetic resonance imaging 25
malpositions 28–9
malpresentations 29
management, of labour 4–7
massage 15
meconium 8, 10, 41, 42
meconium aspiration syndrome 10
membranes, premature rupture 20–3

metoclopramide 13
metronidazole 20, 39
microsampling methods 10
midwifery led units 2
mobile epidural 13
monitoring
   cervix 5–6
   techniques 8
morphia 13
mothers, support for 6–7
multiple pregnancies 30
myometrium 36

naloxone 13, 42
National Birthday Trust 12, 13, 15, 16
nerve blocks 14
newborn, care of 40–3
nimesulide 22
nitrous oxide 12
non-pharmacological methods, pain
   relief 14–15

obstetric emergencies 36–9
occipito-posterior position 28
occipito-transverse position 28–9
O'Driscoll 8, 25
oestrogen 4
operative delivery 31–5
ORACLE 22
oxygen supply 6
oxytocic, stimulation 37
oxytocic drugs 6, 18, 25, 38
oxytocin 5, 30

pain, relief of 12–15
Pain Relief in Labour 12
partners, presence of 8
partograms 5, 24, 25
perinatal mortality 31
perineal tears, degree of severity 35
peritoneum 36
pethidine 12–13, 15
Pfannenstiel's incision 32
pharmacological methods, pain relief
   12–14
phenytoin 26
Philpott, Hugh 5
physiological management 6

physiology
   labour 4–7
   newborn 40
place of birth 1–3
placenta 32, 39, 40
   abruption of 36
   delivery of 6
placenta praevia 17, 31, 36–7
polyhydramnios 22
positive pressure ventilation 41
postmortem examinations 39
postnatal depression 39
postpartum haemorrhage 37–8
postpartum infection 38–9
pre-eclampsia 6, 26, 32
pregnancy
   malpositions 28–9
   malpresentations 29
presentations, unusual 28–30
preterm babies
   conditions and viability 23
   resuscitation 42–3
preterm delivery 22–3
preterm labour
   causes of 20–1
   diagnosis of 21
   management of 21–3
primary postpartum haemorrhage 37–8
progesterone 4
prolapsed umbilical cords 29–30
prostaglandins 5, 16, 18, 19, 36
protease inhibitors 27
proteinuria 26
psychological conditions 39
puerperal psychosis 39
pulmonary circulation 40
pulse oximetry 26

regional blocks 32
relative disproportion 25
relaxation 15
resuscitation, newborn 40–3
rheumatic fever 26
Roberts and Young 16

scalp trauma 34
secondary postpartum haemorrhage 38
selective caesarean delivery 23

shoulder dystocia 9, 30
Silastic caps 34
Simpson's forceps 33
sodium bicarbonate 42
spinal anaesthesia 14
spinal blocks 32
steroids 22, 38
stillbirth 39
subcuticular prolene 32
support, for mothers 6–7
symphysiotomy 30
syntocinon 6, 8, 18, 19
syntometrine 32

tachyphylaxis 21
TENS 15
thrombosis 32
tocolysis 21–2
tocolytics 19, 22, 29
tracheal intubation 40, 41, 42
transverse lie presentation 29
trial of labour 25
trilene 12

umbilical cord, prolapsed 29–30
umbilical venous catheterisation 42
uterine contractions 6, 21, 38
uterine rupture 19
uterine spasm 36
uterus, inversion of 38

vacuum extraction 28
vacuum extractors
   complications 34
   procedure for 34
   types of 34
   use of 34
ventilation 40, 41, 42, 43
ventouse see vacuum extractors
vitamin K 43
volume expanders 42

wave form analysis 10
women centred care 3
Wrigley's forceps 32

zidovudine 27